PRAISE FOR
THE SKY WAS FALLING

"A thoroughly absorbing read: Vividly told, dramatic, goose-bumpy, gripping, and terrifying. Dr. Griggs brings us onto the wards—and into her own mind—as she and her fellow doctors engage in battle against the virus."

—Lesley Stahl, *60 Minutes* correspondent

"Pediatric surgeon Griggs shares her frantic experiences during the first months of the Covid-19 pandemic in this poignant debut memoir . . . Interspersed throughout are gripping passages about performing complicated surgeries on young patients and flashbacks illuminating Griggs's path to becoming a surgeon. Her well-calibrated combination of polemic and personal history will keep readers glued to the page."

—*Publishers Weekly*

"As a doctor who worked through that terrible spring of 2020, I was familiar with the story Cornelia Griggs tells in *The Sky Was Falling*, and yet I tore through this raw and riveting book in one sitting with my heart in my mouth. Unsparingly honest, *The Sky Was Falling* will surely be a classic among the growing body of Covid-19 narratives."

—Suzanne Koven, MD, author of *Letter to a Young Female Physician* and Writer-in-Residence at Massachusetts General Hospital

"In eloquent prose, Dr. Cornelia Griggs recounts her experiences on the front line of the Covid pandemic. Her unique perspective—melding the personal, as a young mother, and the professional, as a skilled doctor—both deeply educates and powerfully elevates the reader. Covid is still with us, and there will be other epidemics in the future. *The Sky Was Falling* is an essential work that provides lasting insights and lessons for the individual and society."

—Jerome Groopman, MD, *New York Times* bestselling author of *How Doctors Think* and Raphael Recanati Professor of Medicine at Harvard Medical School

"This gripping memoir of life during the pandemic inside one of New York's greatest teaching hospitals—NewYork Presbyterian/Columbia Medical Center—is as brave as it is moving. *The Sky Was Falling* has it all—the lack of masks and attempts to censor doctors who spoke out, an ER doctor who took her own life, a legendary transplant surgeon who almost died, and the gladiators of health care who fought to save their beloved city. Griggs's rigor and mission are inspiring."

—Marie Brenner, author of *The Desperate Hours: One Hospital's Fight to Save a City on the Pandemic's Front Lines*

"A recommended purchase . . . a remarkable insider's view . . . This debut author's writing style and fast-paced story will appeal to readers interested in a behind-the-scenes look at hospital operations and personnel during the COVID pandemic."

—*Library Journal*

THE SKY WAS FALLING

FALLING

*A Young Surgeon's Story
of Bravery, Survival, and Hope*

DR. CORNELIA GRIGGS

GALLERY BOOKS

New York   Amsterdam/Antwerp   London   Toronto   Sydney   New Delhi

G

Gallery Books
An Imprint of Simon & Schuster, LLC
1230 Avenue of the Americas
New York, NY 10020

NOTE: Names and identifying characteristics of individuals
have been changed.

First Gallery Books trade paperback edition March 2025

GALLERY BOOKS and colophon are registered trademarks
of Simon & Schuster, LLC

For information about special discounts for bulk purchases, please contact Simon &
Schuster Special Sales at 1-866-506-1949 or business@simonandschuster.com.

The Simon & Schuster Speakers Bureau can bring authors to your live event. For
more information or to book an event, contact the Simon & Schuster Speakers
Bureau at 1-866-248-3049 or visit our website at www.simonspeakers.com.

Interior design by Hope Herr-Cardillo

Manufactured in the United States of America

10 9 8 7 6 5 4 3 2 1

The Library of Congress has cataloged the hardcover edition as follows:

Names: Griggs, Cornelia, author.
Title: The sky was falling : a young surgeon's story of bravery, survival,
   and hope / Dr. Cornelia Griggs.
Description: First Gallery Books hardcover edition. | New York : Gallery
   Books, 2024. | Summary: "The dramatic, cathartic diary of Dr. Cornelia
   Griggs—a young pediatric surgeon and the mother of two toddlers—as
   she worked on the front lines during the first wave of the COVID-19
   pandemic at one of New York City's busiest hospitals"—Provided by
   publisher.
Identifiers: LCCN 2023020393 (print) | LCCN 2023020394 (ebook) | ISBN
   9781982168483 (hardcover) | ISBN 9781982168506 (ebook)
Subjects: LCSH: Griggs, Cornelia. | Pediatric surgeons—New York
   (State)—New York—Biography. | COVID-19 Pandemic, 2020—New York
   (State)—New York—Personal narratives. | COVID-19 Pandemic, 2020—New
   York (State)—New York—Anecdotes. | COVID-19 (Disease)—New York
   (State)—New York.
Classification: LCC RD27.35.G75 A3 2024 (print) | LCC RD27.35.G75 (ebook)
   | DDC 617.092—dc23/eng/20231127
LC record available at https://lccn.loc.gov/2023020393
LC ebook record available at https://lccn.loc.gov/2023020394

ISBN 978-1-9821-6848-3
ISBN 978-1-9821-6849-0 (pbk)
ISBN 978-1-9821-6850-6 (ebook)

For my husband and kids, Rob, Eloise & Jonah.

And to all the "essential workers" of 2020.

AUTHOR'S NOTE

I have intentionally changed details including names, ages, and dates of the patients described in this book to protect their identities. I have also given most of my friends and coworkers pseudonyms. While certain identifying details have been changed or omitted, I will echo the words of physician and author Dr. Michelle Harper: "the human experience at the center of this story is true and unfolded as described." I also intentionally omitted the names of the specific hospitals where I worked to help underscore that this is a story that is representative of many urban U.S. hospitals in 2020.

PREFACE

When I started keeping a detailed diary in February 2020, I was a pediatric surgery fellow at one of New York City's top hospitals in the home stretch of nearly a decade of medical training. I had just signed the contract for my dream job as a full-fledged pediatric surgeon in Boston, where my husband had already begun his own surgical career and was waiting for me and our two young children to join him. Living as a single mom while completing my fellowship already made it a tough time. It soon became unimaginably harder.

What follows is my diary of the next six soul-scorching months. Before pursuing a medical career, I intended to be a journalist, and as the Covid-19 pandemic wrecked my world, I turned to writing as a kind of therapy. I made the time to write at home, usually late at night when I had anxiety-fueled insomnia.

This book details everything I saw and did in those dark and terrifying months inside the walls of a New York City hospital while most of the city was locked down at home. My story is a true-to-life account and a cautionary tale to future generations should they have to face another pandemic. I recognize that many people feel they never want to think or worry about Covid ever again, but this book is about our shared human capacity to survive inconceivable tragedy and trauma. I don't like the saying "What doesn't kill you makes you stronger." I think it all leaves a mark. Yet, I also believe that reflection and recollection can be healing.

There is so much that has already been written about the Covid-19 pandemic, but very few people had the front-row hospital experience that I did. Like so many healthcare workers, I ran to dying patients and performed chest compressions in full personal protective equipment, sweating under the layers of plastic gear while terrified that I might be spraying a deadly virus into my own airway. I operated on the bellies of children whose intestines were mysteriously necrosing and dying from tiny blood clots caused by Covid. Every doctor, nurse, and healthcare worker has their own story to tell. Like me, most of those frontline medical workers were women. Many of them, also like me, were parents and frantically worried about bringing a deadly virus home after a day of treating infected patients. The collective trauma and moral injury suffered by all healthcare workers from that time is still unfolding.

Many colleagues of mine did much more daily, hands-on Covid care than me. As Covid struck, I continued to perform surgeries that were unrelated to the pandemic. Perhaps having some distance from the hourly traumas in the ER and ICU gave me a clearer view of what I saw around me in real time. The shell shock from spending twenty-four-hour days in the Covid ICU wards meant that many of my closest friends and colleagues, in order to survive, had to freeze out or compartmentalize the experiences of those days and erase the painful details from their minds. I took a different approach. I recorded everything because I knew that we were living and working through something historic. I would also soon be leaving for another hospital, which meant I had the luxury to speak up about what I was seeing. This included the unconscionable lack of protective gear for health workers. The gowns and gloves I once threw away without a thought disappeared from our shelves like batteries before a hurricane. I wrote op-eds and went on TV to push for more manufacturing and donation of critical gear. For a time, I became one of the media's "Covid doctors."

After years of surgical training, I developed a reflexive ability to turn off my emotions in order to function at my job. Pre-pandemic, this skill allowed me to whisk dying children from the trauma bay to the operating room, to use blades on their bodies with the decisive and commanding nature required of a surgeon. There's no crying in baseball or surgery. But some things still get through: the haunting sounds of wailing mothers, the screams of babies in pain. In some ways I think my softness and humanity as a young mother is my greatest strength as a pediatric surgeon. When I have a sick patient about the same age as one of my children, I can feel a sudden grip on my throat, a sudden welling up of tears when a child looks up at me with fear as we roll them back to the operating room. It takes a huge effort to disguise my emotions and hold back my impulse to cry. "Don't worry: I promise everything is going to be okay," I say to my patients as I grasp their tiny hands. But I carry it all with me, and once I'm away from the operating room, I have to let it out. Writing helps.

We've all lost something or someone to Covid. Many people have lost parents, grandparents, children, or dear friends. Still more have lost their jobs, their homes, their school years, and the sense of stability that characterized life for many before the pandemic. We lost the easy confidence in our daily routines: home, work, travel, holidays, parties, celebrations. Many of us, myself included, lost our sanity at times. The pandemic has forever planted a nagging uncertainty and danger into the moments of togetherness that bound us in pre-pandemic times. A wet cough is all it takes to put everyone on edge in a crowd.

While I am grateful that I didn't lose a close family member, my house, or my job, like many healthcare workers I lost the illusion that my own life and work were paramount to my employer. In the years since the pandemic started, I have grown more cynical, skeptical, and sometimes despondent about the future of medicine and healthcare, which is increasingly being driven by corporate and financial constraints that make our jobs even more stressful than they need to be. Our nation's hospitals are collapsing from the inside. The consequences of the Covid pandemic are still unfolding. There's a staffing shortage as hundreds of thousands of healthcare workers—including some of my closest friends and mentors—have left the profession they once loved. Nurses are overworked and underpaid, often covering an unsafe number of patients on their shifts. Emergency rooms are overflowing with patients lined up in the hallways. Wait times of more than eight hours have become the new normal. Pediatric wards are shutting down left and right because they don't drive enough revenue to hospitals. And the mental health crisis among our nation's young people has everyone alarmed. If our society can't make sick children a priority, how are we supposed to support and grow the next generation? Healthcare in the United States was broken before Covid, but the pandemic has left even our nation's best hospitals in critical condition.

Despite this bleak outlook on healthcare, the main thing that keeps me coming to the hospital is my belief in the goodness of taking care of sick children. I hope you will see in my stories about my patients that children are both astonishingly fragile and resilient. And if I'm being honest, I am addicted to the dopamine rush of saving young lives. Nothing infuses you with blinding hope quite like bringing a child back from the edge. I want to believe that our nation's hospitals can be resuscitated too. Look at what we've just survived. Last summer I enrolled in a master's program in public health. If another pandemic does happen in my lifetime, I want to be prepared to help steer policies to get it right. For my sanity and for my own children's sake, I believe that there is a possibility to rebuild for the better. I hope these pages help you more fully understand the urgency of this task.

2020

WEDNESDAY, FEBRUARY 19

—

THURSDAY, FEBRUARY 20

Goddamnit. I pull up an X-ray on my laptop. Her lung is down. I have to go back in. I call my resident back. "I'll be there in twenty to thirty. I'm getting in an Uber soon. Set up, please, and get consent from her parents. Thanks." Since I'm the senior pediatric surgery fellow, trips to the hospital in the middle of the night are an exhausting but routine part of my job.

I throw on my down jacket, the one that shields me from the icy, whipping winds of downtown Manhattan in these bleakest of February nights. I tiptoe past my son's crib; he's only two and is practically invisible, buried beneath his loveys and blanket. My four-year-old daughter is soundly sleeping, limbs akimbo. "Baby" has fallen onto the floor next to her. I carefully tuck her back in next to my daughter, who will be looking for that worn-down doll the minute she wakes in the morning. Even though I'm almost never there for that moment, because my normal workday starts before 6:00 a.m., I know this about her.

My Uber arrives in a flash. At this point I have diamond status, with points I can put toward rides or Uber Eats from my frequent trips to the other end of the island, always in the black of night or predawn hours. The twinkling lights of New Jersey smile at me across the Hudson as we cruise up the West Side Highway. The best part of commuting at 3:00 a.m. is the lack of traffic in Manhattan. I'm at the hospital in less than twenty minutes.

My favorite guard is on duty tonight. "What's up, Doc?" he asks with a wink as I enter the lobby. The joke never gets old for us. "Living the dream, Victor, living the dream!" I reply. He knows the punishing hours I work.

Part of what makes these nights bearable is that the end is in sight. After nine years, my medical training will officially be over. It began in New York with medical school and continued with two years of residency in New York, after which I transferred my residency to Boston in order to finish it with my husband. It is now being capped off by a two-year surgical fellowship back at the same hospital in New York where I completed medical school and started my residency. At the end of July, just months from now, I'll be a board-certified attending surgeon.

This last year has been tough. My husband, Rob, also a doctor, started his job as a full-fledged surgeon in Boston, where the kids and

I will join him when I'm done with my fellowship. Could everything *really* be falling into place?

I press the elevator button for the ninth floor, home to our massive pediatric ICU, and rush to the bedside of our sickest patient, Angie, the little girl with the collapsed lung.

"All set for the pigtail?" I ask my team. A pigtail is a small catheter to evacuate air or fluid; in this case I'll be placing the tube into Angie's chest to help re-expand her lung. I review the X-ray and the settings on the extracorporeal membrane oxygenation (ECMO) machine that is doing the breathing for Angie, outside of her little body. The machine pumps and oxygenates a patient's blood, allowing the heart and lungs to rest. It's pretty unusual for a nine-year-old to be on ECMO. It's used when the highest settings on more commonly employed ventilators aren't enough.

I can't believe I have to put another tube in this child, who is just a few years older than my own children. This is her third tube. She has angelic features that fit her name—and the longest eyelashes I've ever seen. Angie's Dominican family has been sitting vigil throughout her entire stay, praying and rocking over her whenever they can.

Angie first came into the hospital with a bad case of pneumonia that got rapidly worse. Whatever virus she caught has damaged her heart function as well as her lungs. Every winter in the worst of cold and flu season we see previously healthy children in the ICU who suddenly get super-sick. The emergent ECMO Angie required as she rapidly deteriorated was scary and unusual enough, but more concerning was the fact that she continued to get worse even then. Usually we can save children from the flu, no matter how severe the case.

The thing is, she doesn't have the flu. She's tested negative for it and every other bug on our viral panels. Viral cardiomyopathy—heart failure caused by a viral illness—is our best guess at a diagnosis at this point. But she's been on ECMO for almost a month already. Her lungs seem to be refusing to get better. She's circling the drain, still alive but showing no signs of improvement.

I'm confident I can at least help her lungs momentarily with the pigtail chest tube. I get on the phone with a translator speaking to her parents, both recent immigrants to the United States. "Whatever you need to do, Doctor," they whisper with deference. I want to embrace them, to cry with them, to hold their pain. But I have an urgent procedure to do.

The chest tube goes in easily with the familiar pop that signals to my knowing hands I'm in the right spot. I've placed hundreds of chest tubes at this point in my training. The repeat X-ray shows that Angie's lung has re-expanded. A slow trickle of old, dark blood drains out the chest tube. Her thick black eyelashes are draped over her eyes. The endotracheal tube and massive swelling around her face obscure how beautiful she really is under the tangle of conduits and wires attached to her body. For tonight, I've helped her stay alive. But this is no way to live. I trudge downstairs to my windowless office to regroup.

It's too late to go home. I have to start rounds again in less than two hours. When I reach my call room I collapse on the cracked and peeling red pleather couch. It's a grotesque specimen that I'm told has been in the fellow's office for over twenty years now, but it's offered me some semblance of sleep for the many nights that I've been called into the hospital. Being "on call," which I am every other night, means being available to return to the hospital to treat patients for emergency care. But I'm unable to sleep. *What the hell is wrong with Angie and why can't her lungs recover?* This is no normal flu.

I switch on the space heater my office mates keep illegally and finally fall asleep. I wake to someone fumbling with the ancient lock of the call room. Victor the security guard must have come by to check on me and then quietly locked the door so no one would disturb me.

Samantha, my junior fellow, enters with her keys in hand and flips on the bright electric lights. She is the younger sister I always wanted but never had. "Oh, shoot, I'm sorry," she mutters when she sees me curled up on the couch. My phone reads 4:59 a.m., a minute away from my alarm. "No, it's fine, I need to get up anyway," I grumble. I have rounds. "Angie needed another chest tube last night," I update her.

"Another one? Shoot," Samantha says.

We make coffee and plop in front of our computers, running through the vitals of our "babies" (as I fondly refer to our patients), scrutinizing the numbers for signs of illness or healing. We take

7

care of the sickest children in the city here, from micro-preemies in the neonatal ICU (NICU) to teenagers with gunshot wounds. And we're both astute clinicians at this stage in our training. Sam and I oversee a team of about six residents and medical students. We've been through seven years of general surgery training already, and this pediatric surgery fellowship is our finishing program. There are only about forty spots a year in pediatric surgery fellowships in the United States (a little less than half of which are at last being filled by women now, after decades of a much greater disparity). At my hospital there are only eight pediatric surgeons in total, fellows included. It's known as the most competitive sub-specialty in general surgery if not all surgery. It will be nearly a decade since medical school graduation before we fellows begin our first "real" jobs out of training, as I'm about to do in Boston. I have done all this for the privilege of operating on babies, despite the brutal work hours of the fellowship, because it's the best and most rewarding job I can imagine.

I see and make plans for dozens of children before 7:30 a.m., when I'm seeing my first "case," meaning the first patient I'm operating on. I quickly update the attending physicians—the supervising doctors who are ultimately in charge of hospital patients' care—and then I'm off to my happy place: the operating room. Room 5 is like my second home now. The ritual and intensity of the operating room have always made me feel safe. Somehow, when I'm operating, I go into an altered state of consciousness, laser focused on the task in front of me. It's been this way since medical school, when I watched my first operation on a patient's carotid artery. Each human being contains a predictable set of organs, but subtle differences make our anatomies as unique as our faces. As a surgeon, you come armed with knowledge and experience with human anatomy and a reverence for the surprises that lie under the skin: the unexpected course of an artery that feeds the liver, an abundance of fat in the overweight, or a paucity of it in a cachectic cancer patient who is wasting away. Every appendectomy is the same but also slightly, sometimes wildly different. And there are always new ways that even the most standard procedures can go wrong.

I tie my lucky scrub cap behind my neck. It's the one that held my hair back when I got a child with cancer out of major aortic bleeding, and the one I wore for my first Kasai procedure, in which we created a passage for bile in a newborn who was born without the right liver ducts.

"Good morning, Sophia!" I chirp at my favorite scrub tech.

"You look tired, Griggsy." She shakes her head at me. Sophia sees past my sunny greetings. She's looked out for me since the first day of my fellowship, stealthily handing me the right instruments to make me look slick in front of my teachers—the senior attending surgeons—and guiding me with the right positioning preferred by each one. "Tired is just my look now, Soph," I crack back at her.

We have a challenging case lined up today: the repair of a congenital diaphragmatic hernia. Through tiny openings and with 3mm instruments, we will repair a giant hole in a newborn's diaphragm.

It's a technically difficult procedure, and I'll be doing the entire case under the supervision of one of my attendings. Though I wouldn't trust myself to drive a car, I can still do my job with the utmost focus. The adrenaline rush of the operating room makes my fatigue disappear. When I'm operating, it's like a switch turns off and with it my basic urges to sleep, pee, eat, or even cry.

The case goes beautifully, and I'm wheeling the baby back to the NICU when my phone goes off. "Can you bring some gloves and masks home from the hospital?" my neighbor Kay texts me. "Uh, okay, I'll see what I can do," I text her back.

We both have been closely following the story of a new, deadly coronavirus in China. I'm not overly worked up about it. It still seems like a disease mostly affecting the elderly in China. Though a Chinese eye doctor who was warning about the outbreak of a SARS-like virus did die in early February, and France has just announced its first death a few days ago. I know Europe will give us the best clues about whether or not this is a real crisis I need to worry about, so I'm in a wait-and-see mode.

I text Kay again, thinking more about her request. Taking supplies from the hospital feels wrong, even though our masks were piled high and bountiful the last time I looked. "Let's just order some masks on Amazon. We don't need to take them from the hospital."

"Okay, I'm stocking up on Tylenol and Motrin too," she replies. It's been a rough winter for parents of toddlers. In the hospital, we've had multiple children in intensive care from a severe flu. At my daughter's nursery school, over half the students are currently out sick, but Eloise is standing strong. The teachers took the remaining healthy kids out for pizza in the West Village on a field trip, since so many of the staff were out too.

Kay is a bit of a hypochondriac, so I'm not surprised that she's worried. But my friends in finance who are paid to assess the effects of bad news on the markets are also completely freaking out about this new coronavirus ripping through China. As with Zika, Ebola, H1N1, and MERS, the headlines are alarming but the threat of pestilence still feels remote, a foreign problem. Except for small pockets of cases, those viruses never meaningfully impacted us on American shores. I have confidence in the systems and infrastructure designed to keep us safe here. I have faith that the CDC knows everything possible about combating pathogens and that our country will be better prepared for a pandemic virus than other parts of the world. New Yorkers, especially those with money, can be prone to hysterics, but that's not my world. My role is to remain levelheaded.

I'm stuck late at the hospital that evening, and as I walk out of the OR, I notice the shelf that we usually keep stocked with masks is looking a little thin. It's merely another inconvenience suffered in a day of many difficulties.

When I finally plop down at my computer, Victor is making his rounds. "You going home soon, Doc?" He nudges me.

"Soon, Victor, soon."

I check Angie's vitals and X-ray. They still look terrible. *Why the hell aren't her resting lungs healing?* I swing by her room and check in with the perfusionist. The perfusionists and respiratory therapists watch over our ECMO patients at the bedside 24/7. They are some of the smartest and best teammates I have in the hospital. Usually they are the only reason I can go home at night. Tonight it's Erin on call. She's one of the best on the team—and the funniest.

"How's she doing?" I ask.

"Stably terrible. But nothing we can do about it tonight."

I nod and wince in acknowledgment. We both know Angie is getting worse, despite our best treatment and support. *Enough for today,* I tell myself. And I begin the cold, long trudge home on the subway.

2006–2011

When I first decided to apply to medical school, I had grand visions of becoming a do-it-all family practitioner. I wanted to treat entire families, to deliver babies and watch them suck in their first breaths, to hold the hands of withering octogenarians as they slipped away into a comfortable peace. I wrote an essay extolling the virtues of the family practice and won a small award my first year of medical school that further fueled my idealistic vision.

During my training in the clinics of Washington Heights in upper Manhattan, this wasn't what I usually saw. I watched frazzled primary care physicians rush from room to room, trying to treat patients with uncontrolled diabetes, hypertension, coronary artery disease, asthma, depression, and obesity in hurried fifteen-minute appointments that really required an hour or more.

"You've got to try to tackle just one thing at a time each visit, or else it's too demoralizing," Dr. Murphy warned me while typing her notes between sips of black Café Bustelo coffee. She was only forty years old but already looked sixty, with wiry, untamed salt-and-pepper hair thrown haphazardly into a messy bun at the nape of her neck. She spoke and carried herself in a weary, defeated posture that conveyed the years she had spent battling insurers, putting out fires, and generally doing the job of five different doctors for the pay of less than one. She had already put in her notice that she was moving to North Carolina come summer.

Primary care was nothing like what I imagined. Those clinics laid bare the vast injustices of the United States healthcare system, which indiscriminately reward high-cost, invasive treatments over preventive care. Politically, I still wanted to fight the good fight in the trenches of those clinics. But I could see that I was not temperamentally suited for family medicine or primary care. I was too impatient. I wanted to see results faster. So I tried my hand at neurology, obstetrics, emergency medicine, cardiology, and other specialties.

"I feel like I'm speaking to a cardiologist," the clerkship director told me at the end of my cardiology rotation.

"You will fit right in the club," an obstetrics resident told me as she slung an arm around my shoulders after a twelve-hour overnight shift where we delivered four babies together.

By the end of my third year, I felt like I had tried to belong everywhere but still hadn't found my home.

Surgery was the most notoriously difficult rotation in medical school. Medical students aiming to become surgeons would routinely make their rounds at the hospital at 4:30 a.m. to draw blood and collect the patient data for the day. And the competition was cutthroat. More than a third of my class wanted to go into a surgical specialty of some sort. Our school was known for churning out highly trained neurosurgeons and orthopedic surgeons with Abercrombie model looks. I wasn't interested in elbowing my classmates out of the way for a space at the operating table.

When it came time for my surgery rotation, I chose an assignment upstate in Cooperstown, New York, where my school had an affiliation with a local community hospital. Medical students would stay in a house owned by the medical school and live dorm-style with a family supper at the dining room table every night. I chose the rotation mostly because I needed a break from New York City and some time to plan my next move. I had to make a decision about residency in the next three months or else take a gap year to do research and buy more time. I hoped the air upstate would clear my lungs and my head.

I packed a duffel and headed to Cooperstown. I sauntered up to rounds at the leisurely hour of 6:00 a.m. that Monday and was met by a friendly second-year resident named Arun.

"Welcome to surgery!" he said, smiling at me. "Here's your assignment for the day. You'll be in the vascular room, helping Dr. K."

The schedule showed my name next to the carotid endarterectomy, a procedure in which the surgeon scrapes plaque out of the carotid artery to prevent future strokes and clots.

"Are you sure he won't mind having a medical student assist?" I asked.

"Not at all. The surgeons here love teaching," Arun assured me.

What I saw in the operating room that day changed my life. Dr. K.'s hands moved like music. He deftly cut open the patient's neck, revealing the glistening blood vessels just beneath the surface. "There's the hypoglossal nerve, and the bifurcation," he pointed out gently as I followed his hands with a suction catheter, sucking up small pools of blood. It was like watching my anatomy textbook come to life in front of me—the Technicolor *Wizard of Oz* moment I could never unsee. I gasped when he applied the clamps to the carotid artery, briefly stopping the blood flow to one side of the brain, then carved out what looked like a hardened chunk of Brie cheese from the patient's artery and closed the hole with a small patch and the tiniest sutures I'd ever seen.

"How long will the patient have to stay in the hospital?" I asked when we were finished with the procedure, which took under two hours. "Oh, he'll go home tomorrow." Dr. K. laughed. My mind was blown. Surgery was the most incredible thing I'd ever witnessed. Dr. K. recognized the combination of hunger and awe in my eyes immediately. "Go get a snack, Griggsy," he chuckled. "We've got an abdominal aortic aneurysm to do next."

My eyes widened. A "triple-A" repair was one of the biggest, scariest operations I could imagine. Medical students weren't even allowed in the room for those repairs at my medical school's main hospital in the city. That was a fellow-level case. But over the course of the next eight hours I found myself tugging and retracting for Dr. K. I felt a rush of pure awe as he placed a graft in the patient's aorta, delicately and swiftly moving his clamps to protect the patient's kidneys. It was like he was following some invisible map he knew instinctively, like when you drive between work and home without even having to turn on your brain. The synchronicity of his hands and instruments was automatic, programmed, but also fluid and mesmerizing.

"If we damaged that branch there," Dr. K. said, pointing to a vessel winding out from the aorta, "the patient could be paralyzed.

"Don't look so scared." Dr. K. laughed. "We're almost done."

When the operation finished, I was officially hooked.

"I think I want to go into surgery," I told my mother over the phone that evening.

"You say that about every rotation," she retorted, surprised at this new change in career trajectory.

"Today was the coolest, best day of medical school by far!" I protested.

"Well, let's see how you feel at the end of the month," she said. My parents were coming to visit me for the holidays and to check out Cooperstown's Baseball Hall of Fame, a bucket list item of theirs.

By the time of their visit, I was even more determined about surgery. After being in the operating room, I could no longer imagine practicing medicine anywhere else. I loved the instant gratification of a successful operation. I loved assisting the surgeons in ushering patients from the brink of death back to life. I loved the adrenaline in the trauma bay, the sense of importance and urgency of the job. I loved sweeping into a code (a cardiac arrest) to place a catheter and inject a lifesaving dose of epinephrine. I even loved the gory parts: a rush of pus from a decompressed abscess, the smell of the burnt flesh from a "Bovie" (an electrosurgical device to cauterize tissue), chopping off a necrotic toe. None of it bothered me. I was addicted, totally.

I was also terrified. I didn't know how or with whom, but I knew for certain that I wanted children someday. I wasn't sure how to reconcile this with my aspirations for surgery. Everything I knew about the life of a surgeon told me it would be all-encompassing, one reason why relatively few women planning a family chose it. While women constituted more than 65 percent of the healthcare workforce at the time, about 80 percent of surgeons were men.

"If you do surgery, you won't be able to have children until your forties at the soonest!" my friend Hadi warned when I got back to the city from Cooperstown. "And your ovaries will probably be shriveled and fried by then," he teased.

"That's fucking harsh!" I razzed him back. Hadi was going to be a cardiologist. He was one of the social chairs with me at med school. We planned most of the post-exam parties for our class.

"Why should I have to choose between the field I love the most and having a family?" I complained. It seemed wholly unfair. It was 2008 and still five years before the terms "lean in" and "girlboss" would enter the millennial professional vocabulary. But I had the aching sense that I wanted to "have it all." I balked at the idea that my professional ambitions needed to be tempered by my desires for a loving relationship and children. I attended seminars for women in medicine where the messaging stressed the need for "balance." At one of these events, a pediatrician said that one of the reasons she had chosen the specialty was that it gave her the ability to have a nice "lifestyle."

"I have three kids and want to be able to pick them up from school every day," she said. "Pediatrics allows me the flexibility to work part-time." The other women panelists nodded their heads. A dermatologist echoed the need for balance. "I need to work out every day," she said. Her toned calves, accentuated by red-bottomed stilettos on her feet, confirmed her dedication to fitness. "I like to have 'me' time, and dermatology lets me have a great balance between work and play." There wasn't a single woman surgeon on the panel.

Finally, the hospital's busiest interventional gastroenterologist took the microphone. "When you're in a procedural field, you often get called away in the middle of the night. You have to ask yourself some hard questions about what that means over the course of a lifetime when deciding on a specialty," she advised. "If you think you want to become a surgeon, you have to ask yourself, 'Is there *any* other field that would make me as happy?' If the answer is yes, don't choose surgery. The personal sacrifices are enormous."

I walked away from the evening crestfallen. The women on the panel had only confirmed the old medical school lore of what was referred to as the "ROAD to success": radiology, ophthalmology, anesthesiology, or dermatology—the "lifestyle-friendly" fields with good pay and limited hours. What I thought would be a night of empowerment seemed to be a humbling warning instead.

At home I thought more deeply about the meaning of "balance." I had never lived my life in balance. It wasn't in my personality. Whatever I was doing, whether it was cramming for a medical school exam, assisting in surgery, or sweating it out on a dance floor in the East Village, I was doing it to the max, with my whole being. I was also stupidly competitive.

Sometimes my habit of taking on too much, of being too intense, would catch up with me. Every six or seven weeks I would crash and sleep until noon and then be a sloth for twenty-four hours, usually after a big exam. Then I would pick myself up and throw myself into the next challenge. When I planned trips, I would bop between cities like I was collecting trophies. Maybe I was a walking cliché of FOMO or had a touch of hypomania, but I generally seemed to have more energy than my peers. Surgery also seemed, well, badass. That was part of the allure too.

How hard could the residency really be?

I was aware that the very hubris of that thought wasn't the worst quality for a surgeon. You had to have a streak of it to brandish a knife for a living. I often think about the fact that, outside of the context of the operating room and medical field, what we do to other human bodies would be considered assault. Maybe it's more than hubris. Maybe every surgeon is somehow a little sick in the head.

So, after thinking it through, I recognized I was just arrogant, naïve, and hungry enough to want it. Dr. Griggs. Surgeon. Maybe I'd even invent a maneuver someday. The Griggs maneuver. It sounded good. Later in residency I would learn that maneuvers were often jokingly named for you when you made a massive and humiliating fuckup in the operating room. My good friend got his procedural moniker when one of his suturing instruments got stuck in someone's pancreas. Now that surgeon always begins his cases with a "Goldstein" stitch to form a protective barrier against errant objects. Surgeons make weird jokes. But even the crude humor and brusque demeanor of the surgical residents enticed me. I wanted into the club. Children or not, I had to go for it. Plus, marriage and children were nowhere on the horizon for me yet. I'd had a string of serious boyfriends in medical school but none of them felt like a soul mate. The guy I was dating at the time certainly wasn't up for being married to a surgeon. He was a workaholic himself; we were compatible because neither of us was needy. We let the other work nonstop and told ourselves the hustle would be worth it someday. I wasn't going to make a career choice based on a life I didn't have. Against conventional wisdom, I decided to apply to surgical residency.

SUNDAY, FEBRUARY 23

—

MONDAY, FEBRUARY 24

It's a Sunday and I've done one big case and two appendectomies by 2:00 p.m. and all I want to do is collapse. I haven't slept a wink this weekend, but I catch the subway to meet my kids and my in-laws, who are looking after them, at the Central Park Zoo. I scroll through Twitter on the train. The stories are alarming. Italy is having a major coronavirus outbreak. There's also buzzing about a possible case in California and an outbreak at a Washington State nursing home. We don't even have a way to test at the hospital. I can't worry about this now. I hop off the train at Fifty-Ninth Street and head toward the zoo. The park is packed. It's a surprisingly warm and sunny day for late February.

The kids haven't seen much of me lately and they start acting out as soon as I arrive. "Hey, guys!" I hug them both tightly in front of the sea lion. My father-in-law looks exasperated and is holding two tote bags, the kids' puffer jackets, and two water bottles while trying to push our squeaky stroller. "Thank God you're here," he says, and smiles wearily.

"Wow, look at the whiskers on that sea lion," I say as I try to lift Jonah up to see them, but he fights and kicks me hard in the gut.

"No *want* to," he protests.

It's going to be that kind of an outing.

"Sweetie, aren't you cold without your jacket?" I ask Eloise.

"*NO!* I don't like that jacket, only the pink one."

They're both wired, hungry, and nobody has napped. There are mobs of harried parents and whining toddlers blocking the view at every exhibit. I reach deep for my last ounce of patience when Eloise collapses onto the ground in the middle of a crowded walkway in front of the polar bears and wails out of nowhere, "I miss Daddy!"

Me too, honey, I think. *Me too.* I desperately wish he could be here to help. I'm hurt and deflated because the one hour I have to be with my kids has dissolved into a fit of toddler tantrums. When I started my fellowship, my son was only six weeks old and I had to find a way to pump breast milk between long cases in the operating room. I've lost over thirty pounds in fellowship from the sheer stress of it all, even though I never seem to find the time to exercise anymore. Still, my arms are strong from carrying my babies and from the long hours in the operating room.

This weekend the chair of the pediatric surgery department asked me where I would like to have my graduation party. The end of this brutal life in surgical training is starting to feel within reach.

My friends who have graduated have bought their dream homes and finally have time to be there for their kids and families. I conjure a future image of myself: I'm looking put together, dropping off my kids at school in Boston. At long last, their teachers will have seen me enough to remember my name. Then I'll head into the hospital for a full day of clinic or cases. On most nights I'll make it home for family dinner, or at least to read to the kids and put them to sleep. This could be my reality in a few short months. What I know for a fact is that I will be on call only one-tenth as often as now and my salary will go up by 500 percent.

We flee the overcrowded park. As I buckle my daughter into her car seat, I notice a faint pink swelling around her eye. Not another illness. Their sheets are already stained from the sticky, sweet syringes of red Tylenol I've been forcing down their gullets to treat the fevers that have been plaguing them nightly for what seems like the past three weeks.

"Does your eye hurt, sweetie?" I ask Eloise.

"Kinda," she says, shrugging.

We head back home to the apartment downtown where I, the kids, my mother, and our golden retriever, Magic, are all currently living, packed into two bedrooms. My parents own the apartment but rarely used it before, and when Rob left for Boston, my mother moved in with me to help out with the kids. Under the bathroom light I take a closer look at Eloise's left eye and, sure enough, it looks like a raging case of pink eye. I call her pediatrician to get a prescription for drops and disinfect all the surfaces in the apartment. I cannot afford to get sick this week. I have the biggest case of my fellowship coming up: separating conjoined twins.

The only other person who really gets it—the impossibility of juggling my mom role with a surgeon's schedule—is Jane, my best friend at work, who is also a pediatric surgeon and the mother of two young kids. We became inseparable as co-fellows together, her the senior to my junior, and now she is technically my boss, as she's in her first year as an attending. I was ecstatic when they hired her and she decided to stay at the hospital after her fellowship. Jane stands five feet tall on a good day and is the definition of a spitfire. She's from Chicago and swears like a sailor—but is also unabashedly girly. Our kids are friends, and we take care of each other. Jane always has my back, and if she hadn't been my senior fellow, I'm not sure I would have survived my first year. We've spent so much time together over the last year and a half that our minds have practically melded. We could be twins if it weren't for the fact that when we operate together, she needs to stand on two stacked stools to make up our height difference.

Last week, when we had to do a colon resection together for a particularly gnarly case of dead bowel, we made the OR team listen to the latest Taylor Swift album three times in a row. The anesthesia team grumbled nearly the whole time but we had a blast: our cheesy music taste is part of our bond. I always make fun of Jane for being "basic" because she likes drinking pumpkin spice lattes, living in leggings, and buying notebooks with sayings like "Live, laugh, love" or "Though she be little, she is fierce." If you didn't know that Jane was a badass surgeon, you could mistake her for a millennial mom cliché. But we both love that we don't have to pretend to be cool for each other.

Having Jane around makes work not only tolerable but fun.

"Do you think we need to be worried?" I ask her as I deliver Starbucks to her office when I come to work on Monday and collapse on her couch. "Are you stockpiling masks and gloves and toilet paper and Tylenol?" I don't have to worry about seeming unsure in front of Jane.

"Why would I stockpile that stuff?" she says, looking puzzled.

"You know, the coronavirus. It looks like it's getting bad in Europe now . . ." I trail off.

"I can't even handle *you* now, Griggs! I can't think about anything except boards." She shakes her frazzled head at me. Lately, she's been consumed with studying for the big test to certify her as a pediatric surgeon.

"Fine," I reply. "I'll just order stuff for you."

Just a week earlier I thought my neighbor Kay was crazy for stockpiling supplies. But now it seems smart, just in case. The frenzy is getting to my head. I know a few ER doctors who have a doomsday prep kit at home. I have a basic first aid kit and a small amount of emergency supplies, but New York City apartments generally aren't conducive to stockpiling. A vision of me setting up a makeshift emergency ward in my living room flashes across my mind. I open the Amazon app to order some basic fluids and IV start kits. Best-case scenario: Kay and I will laugh at ourselves in a few weeks' time for having fallen down this rabbit hole.

On the way home, I refill Eloise's eyedrops. At the pharmacy I suddenly remember the eye doctor from China. The whistleblower for coronavirus. He had noticed many sick patients with conjunctivitis dying from atypical pneumonias before he died from the mysterious disease himself. "Couldn't be . . ." I silence the anxiety building in my mind. I've got to rest for a big week ahead.

SATURDAY, FEBRUARY 29

This will be my second time in the OR witnessing the separation of conjoined twins—usually a once-in-a-lifetime scenario for a pediatric surgeon. The first was back in residency. For fourteen hours I watched the complex reconstruction and was left dazzled by the expertise displayed by the surgeons on the team. The moment when the twins were safely separated felt miraculous, like witnessing a rebirth, and sealed my career choice in pediatric surgery. I decided it was what I needed to do, no matter what.

Now I'm scrubbing in for another pair of conjoined twins, two five-month-old girls, their tiny bodies locked in a face-to-face embrace by a fused abdomen and chest. I've been selected for the team, and this time I expect to get the chance to be an active contributor. Our task today is to separate their hearts and liver, leaving the arteries that are critical for blood supply, and the ducts that would allow both sets of organs to thrive independently. The choreography of the operating room requires us to duplicate our setup at the moment of separation, moving from one operating table to two. If all goes well, it's at that point that I'll become first assistant on one of the teams, helping with the onerous task of closing one of the girls' abdomens and chests.

Dr. O. is the lead surgeon on the case and, after completing the separation, will take charge of the other team. At fifty-five years old, he is one of the hospital's most famous names, a pioneer in transplant surgery, so skilled that he was the first surgeon to transplant six organs into a patient simultaneously. He is our Superman, someone who can operate for more than twenty-four hours at a time without taking a break. Now these two little babies depend on him. Until we open them up, we really won't know whether the operation can succeed and give them both the chance for a normal life. There are all sorts of ethical quandaries, including the risk that one twin, probably the smaller one, could have disastrous bleeding during surgery. It isn't clear that we will safely be able to close both of their bellies after cutting them apart.

But the surgical separation proceeds seamlessly. All of our preparation and teamwork has paid off. As we stare down at the last piece of tissue bridging them, Dr. O. instructs me to make the final cut that will give each of these tiny girls an independent life. It's a kind and generous gesture. I have only a few seconds to process the thrill that pulses through my body as I complete the separation of their bodies. Like an elegant ballet, the team splits into two. Mine carefully lifts one twin away from her sister and goes off to a second operating table. We close our twin's belly, making flaps to allow for the inevitable postoperative swelling. Then we close the layers over her tiny heart and diaphragm. I wonder if she will feel lonely when she wakes up in her own room in the ICU, apart from her sister for the first time in her life.

When I scrub out, I check my work phone to find fifty unread texts. Upstairs, Angie, our ECMO patient, is bleeding out of her chest tube. I race up five flights of stairs to her bedside. The blood is pouring out of her chest and there are ten people in her room. Her blood pressure has dropped so low that she could die. "We've got to do a thoracotomy and get to the source," I bark. "Call the OR and get the thoracotomy tray. And get Jane." I begin prepping her chest with iodine and Jane arrives and scrubs in. The OR team arrives and in less than two minutes Jane and I are in Angie's right chest. It's a disaster. Her lung is blackened, both parts rock-hard and crumbling and bleeding from every surface imaginable. We explore her chest for a fixable injury, but there is no evidence of a vessel tear. It's her entire lung exploding, and all we can do is place sterile packs to try to control the bleeding with direct pressure. Miraculously, the packing temporarily stabilizes her and we put a temporary dressing over her chest.

"Live to fight another day" is sometimes the best outcome you can get in a disaster surgery patient, especially one who has just almost bled to death.

Jane looks at me when we are safely back in her office. "What the hell was that?"

"I don't know," I say. Angie is the same age as Jane's son, Jayden. I can tell she's shaken. Whenever we walk by Angie's room, her

31

mother is always holding her daughter's hand, rocking and pray-ing. Sometimes I can hear her quietly weeping. I understand the unbearable fear and uncertainty weighing on her.

Surgeons are known for their gruffness and hauteur. I haven't picked up these traits and never intend to. I view my empathy as an asset. It helps, I think, that I've recently gone through the experience of having someone I love attached to machines and going through a health crisis that has no promise of a positive outcome. I have some sense of what my patients and their families are feeling.

2014

My pager goes off in the late afternoon on a bitterly cold day in December. I'm in Boston, in my third year of my residency in general surgery.

"68942. Johannes."

The most ominous pages are always brief. I have no idea why Johannes, my favorite chief resident—the group that oversees our schedules and helps with our training—is paging me. We're not even working at the same hospital today. I'm out in the fancy suburbs at an affiliate hospital, my first day on the surgical team there.

As I dial the extension on my pager, I prepare myself for a "beat." A beat is the verbal lashing administered by a senior resident or attending when you screw up, especially in the "Pit," our nickname for the emergency department at the main hospital downtown, where I just finished a month-long stint. Our trauma rotation is notoriously the hardest one of the third year in general surgery. Every other day we spend twenty-four solid hours fielding the sickest surgical patients and traumas that come through the doors. Few people would question that it's the most stressful job in the hospital. I figure I must have screwed something up and Johannes is calling to let me have it. It must be bad if he's bothering to page me now. At least it's Johannes. I respect the hell out of him.

Johannes picks up the phone. "Cornelia, I'm with Rob and I've just checked him into Acute Bay 10. He has a terrible headache. He's acting delirious and talking nonsense. It's not an emergency, but is there any way for you to get here? He's going to get a CT scan."

Instead of feeling terrified, I'm relieved. Rob having a headache is better than me having made a giant mistake in the Pit, isn't it?

"Of course," I answer. "I'll be right over."

Rob, my husband, is also a third-year surgery resident in our program. We've been texting all day about how crappy we both feel. After the nearly sleepless month in the Pit, I've come down with a soupy cold and constant nausea. It didn't surprise me when Rob sent me a text around 11:00 a.m. to say that he felt terrible too.

"I feel very sick," he'd told me. "Nauseated. Sweaty."

It was exactly how I'd been feeling, so I told him, "I'm sorry, baby . . . I'm sure we have the same thing. I'm so sorry . . . I gave it to you."

I gather my things and say goodbye to the rest of the surgery team at the affiliate hospital. It's a big deal for me to leave, but I tell them that Rob is in the ED and I've got to figure out what is going on. I even joke with them: I've managed to tough out a long day of operating with the same cold. "Dudes—they can't even handle a common cold!" I laugh as I leave the surgical ward.

When I pull out of the hospital parking lot, I get a call from Rob. He's crying. In between big, sobbing gulps he says something I can't even begin to believe. "I have a tumor. My brain is rotting." I can barely understand him. I tell him to breathe. I tell him he's not making sense. I'm on my way and will be there in fifteen minutes. He begs me to come fast.

At this point I can't tell if Rob is truly delirious over the phone. The comment about his brain "rotting" doesn't sound like him, since he's a stickler about medical terminology. He must have a fever or some kind of infection that is causing him to speak irrationally. Rob is the smartest resident in our class of über-achievers. He's a walking medical encyclopedia and always has the right answers. We joke that it's as if a divine power intervenes when he's taking a test, because he's never scored below the 98th percentile on anything, whether or not he studies. The truth is he's just a medical genius, which makes being married to him both wonderful and occasionally infuriating.

As I'm driving toward the hospital downtown I can feel myself shifting into crisis mode: my armor is on and I'm laser focused on the task in front of me, hyperaware of all my surroundings. I may be only a resident, but the transition into this mode is seamless for me now. I spend so many of my days working and living in the middle of life-and-death crises and know by now that I thrive in this zone. Usually when I'm in it, I'm dealing with crises that are not my own. When a patient with a gunshot wound or a burn victim comes through the door, it's not my flesh on fire. This is different. Rob is my world. I expect to find my mind churning with terrified thoughts. My husband has just told me that he has a brain tumor. Instead, the same familiar calm comes over me.

I lock the car and sprint to the emergency department. Rob is in the "acute" area of the ED, which is where they put the sickest patients. I'm starting to accept that something is deeply, horribly wrong. When I get to Rob's room, the lights are off and the door is closed. I slide the door open and see Rob's face, pale and bloated with tears.

Rob starts crying again, but this time he's perfectly clear. "They did a CT scan and there's a five-centimeter mass in my brain." I look over at the computer and the image is sitting right there on the screen. Surgeons need to see to believe, and the screen tells the awful proof. I scroll through the images of my husband's brain—the brain that convinced him to love me, to marry me. A clementine-sized circle engulfs much of the left side of his brain. It's so big that it has shifted his brain matter across the midline, a deadly sign in some of our trauma patients. I jump onto his hospital stretcher and hold him. I coo soothing words into his ear and run my fingers through his hair, now damp with sweat. I tell him that whatever it is, we're going to get through it together—that I love him more than anything and I know it's going to be okay. We'll fight it together. I actually hate the "fighter" metaphor with cancer but I can't think of anything better to say at that moment. The truth is you don't so much fight cancer as you make a truce with it.

We're still sitting together in the dark when Mindy, a neurology resident, comes into the room. She worked as Rob's intern when he was the senior resident on the pediatric surgery team, and now she's the one who's been called to consult on him as a patient in the ED. As Mindy explains what we already know—that they've found a 5cm mass in Rob's brain—I see a look in her eyes that will become familiar to me over the next few weeks. There's a palpable timidity that overcomes the residents who are taking care of Rob, cutting through their usual confidence and clarity. It's terrifying and destabilizing to treat one of your own. Medical training is a long-term investment and full of personal sacrifice. Early mortality is not supposed to be part of the bargain.

Mindy begins to get choked up. "I've asked Dr. Plotkin to come see you. He's the absolute best neuro-oncologist in the hospital. If it were my . . ." Mindy swallows and trails off.

"Thank you so much, Mindy," I say, stopping her. "We really appreciate it." I'm playing the protective wife role. I want to shield Rob from the pity and the pain that is so obvious on her face. I also want to show Mindy that we're not going to live up to the worst version of the reputation of surgical residents at the hospital. For decades our program was considered "malignant," a blanket term in medical culture for *hostile*. Our reputation has softened with work-hour restrictions and a focused effort on culture change, but some surgery residents still have a habit of degrading the medical residents like Mindy and even of sleeping with the nurses in on-call rooms, barking orders at the junior residents—fitting the old-school stereotype of surgeon-lotharios.

———

We learn that the mass in Rob's brain is a nasty tumor called an anaplastic astrocytoma—a high-grade glioma with poor survival rates. Over the next few months, Mindy, her medicine colleagues, the surgeons, and everyone else taking care of Rob prove themselves to be incredibly capable physicians. Rob receives the best possible surgical and cancer follow-up treatment, including radiation and later chemo. He remains tough, an innate quality of his. He even continues to find ways to make me and the other people around him laugh when it feels like the world is ending.

The anesthesia team that took care of him during the removal of his brain tumor was amazed that he had the wherewithal to crack jokes during surgery. To ensure critical language and speech areas of his brain would not be injured, a large portion of his tumor removal procedure was done while he was awake under MRI guidance. As the neurosurgeons chipped away at the tumor in his brain, the OR team would quiz him and show him pictures of barnyard animals. Holding up a picture of a pig, they asked him to name the animal. "Not kosher," Rob answered with a smile.

In less than ten months from the time of his diagnosis, Rob is back in the operating room. He will have an MRI of his brain every six months, indefinitely, as there is always the risk of recurrence with his type of brain tumor. After each one, we hold our breaths for twenty-four hours until the neuro-oncologist calls with the results. The silver lining is that, in a world in which future crises are inevitable, we discover our ability to come to terms with the uncertainty of life.

MONDAY, MARCH 2
—
TUESDAY, MARCH 3

It's an uncharacteristically slow morning, so after grabbing Starbucks for the team I sit down to check the news at my desk. "A second person has died of the novel coronavirus in the Seattle area and more confirmed cases of the illness have emerged in Washington State, officials said Sunday evening." The stock market has been gyrating wildly all week.

I can feel this coronavirus closing in on us in New York. An outbreak now feels inevitable. Twitter posts by public health experts are pointing out that, with our swarming airports, packed subways, and densely crowded neighborhoods, New York City is prime real estate for a viral pandemic. I've got to get off social media. I'm becoming paranoid and I need to stay focused at work.

I can't stop myself from wondering if it's possible that Covid is already here, though. I think back to that week when only two kids were healthy enough to attend Eloise's class. For most of February it felt like every kid I met had a cough. And I've started to wonder out loud to Corinne, our ECMO fellow, whether Covid might explain why Angie's lungs can't seem to recover. The pediatric ICU (PICU) team decided to test her this week. We now have the ability to take test samples and send them out to a city-wide lab. But the results came back negative. Still, I'm not sure how reliable the tests can be when we seem to know so little about the way this virus behaves.

There's a knock at my office door and Jamie, one of our physician assistants, pokes her head in. "The ED just paged: there's a teenager downstairs with spontaneous pneumothorax."

"Stable?" I ask.

"Totally," she says.

"Okay, good. Let's go down and check and we can set up for a tube."

It seems like I'm putting in chest tubes every damn day lately. But at least this one is a run-of-the-mill spontaneous pneumo-thorax, which is common and tends to happen in tall, slim teenagers. Bubbles at the tops of their lungs can develop, called blebs. When this happens, they are prone to having their lungs drop and usually require a chest tube and sometimes a simple operation to get the lung back up.

Jamie and I walk down to the ED and start grabbing supplies. When we get to the door of the patient's room, there is a big yellow sign on the door that says: RESPIRATORY PRECAUTIONS.

"What is this?" I ask Jamie. "The ED put her on Covid precautions because she was coughing? Seriously?"

Jamie shrugs at me. "They must have just put that sign up. It wasn't here when I first came down," she says as she begins to don the gown and gloves required to enter the room.

The kid has a pneumo. Of course she's coughing, I think. The patient has no fever or any other signs suggestive of infection. I've brushed up on the limited literature that's out there so far about treatment protocols for Covid. The imaging findings on chest X-rays and CT scans are pretty classic: we look for something called opacities or consolidations in the lungs. I double-check the kid's chest X-ray on a nearby computer. Her lungs look clear. The ED is probably overreacting to this case, I figure. Putting this kid on precautions seems unnecessary and reactionary to me. Looks like I'm not the only paranoid one.

Jamie and I go behind the ED desk and grab two duckbills, the colloquial name for the orange-and-white hospital-issued N95 masks. They, along with the standard, simple surgical masks, used to be easily findable on open shelving but now are stored—or guarded—at the front of each department and we have to ask for them. There's a clipboard outside the patient's room and the ED asks us to sign our names and employee ID numbers before we enter. I gear up with a paper gown and gloves and then layer a surgical mask over the N95. We've been told to try to reuse the N95s if possible, which seems sort of disgusting. Typically, an N95 is something I'd throw away after one use. Hopefully there's a big shipment for restocks on the way. I slide open the door and a whoosh of air gets sucked into the room from the negative pressure system.

"Hi there. I'm Dr. Griggs, the senior pediatric surgery fellow. I've reviewed your chest X-ray and there is a collapse of your right lung. We're going to need to place a tiny chest tube to help the lung re-expand."

I walk the family through the risks and benefits of the procedure and set up for the tube. Hopefully she'll need a chest tube for only a short time and then be on her way home. I numb the skin over her ribs, place a needle in her chest until I get a rush of air into my syringe, slide a small wire into her chest through the needle, and then swiftly advance the chest tube up along the wire. The tube slips in easily and the whole procedure takes less than five minutes. The patient coughs loudly for several minutes as her lung expands. Coughing after a chest tube placement is very normal. But I catch myself holding my breath anyway. I secure the chest tube with a dressing and reassure the patient that everything looks good and like classic spontaneous pneumothorax in every way. Still, I get out of the room as quickly as possible.

I document on the clipboard the amount of time I spent in the room. Fifteen minutes total.

"Well, that was weird," I say to Jamie.

She's being uncharacteristically quiet. "Yeah. It feels like I can barely breathe in those masks," she says.

"At least it was an easy tube," I say with a shrug. Then I'm off to the next patient.

I walk upstairs from the ED to the operating room. Just a full schedule of simple elective cases today. For once, my list of things to do seems manageable. Upstairs, the separated twins are healing wonderfully from their procedure. The day goes smoothly and no major disasters present themselves.

But the next day, when I'm at home on a rare day off, Jamie texts me and then calls me, which she only does in an emergency. "The chest tube kid from yesterday—she's positive for coronavirus."

"You're kidding me," I say.

"I wish I was." She sighs.

"Well, what do we do now?"

"The infection control person says it's fine because we were wearing the masks."

"Thank God we did."

"Yeah, I guess."

"Do we need to get tested?"

"She said no unless we get symptoms," Jaime responds.

Suddenly I'm replaying the last twenty-four hours in sequence. Eloise had trouble falling asleep last night, so I climbed into her bed to rub her back. As I always do, I briefly fell asleep in her bed before being awakened by her tossing and kicking. Eloise has always been a good sleeper, but she kicks like crazy, so I can never stay there long. When I woke up at midnight to drag myself back to my own room, I leaned over the crib and kissed Jonah on his cheek. He still sleeps in a baby position with his tush straight up in the air. Wait: now that I think of it, I gave Jonah a bite of my sushi last night. He thinks it's hilarious and loves the taste of sticky rice. Holy shit. If I got coronavirus from the teenager, my kids are definitely infected.

I call Jane.

"This shit just got real."

"What happened?"

"I put a chest tube in a kid yesterday and she's positive. But she wasn't having any symptoms."

"Just calm down. It's probably fine," Jane reassures me.

"I guess I'll know soon." I laugh. What else can I do.

"Griggs, you're fine," Jane repeats.

"Yeah, I know. This just sucks."

"Hopefully it'll be over soon," she says.

I hang up and am suddenly overcome with a terrifying feeling of powerlessness. If I infected Eloise and Jonah, I'll never forgive myself. They've already lost so much of me to this job. I've given up so many moments with them and I always rationalize by telling myself it's harder on me than it is on them. They won't remember that I missed Jonah's first steps. They won't remember me leaving silently in the middle of the night while they slept. But now Covid makes the stakes feel higher. Is being here for other people's children worth it if it means infecting my own? Luckily, I don't have much time to ponder the answer, because my phone lights up with a call from the ICU.

Later that day the president declares a national emergency.

"They're talking about setting up drive-through testing all across the nation," my mom tells me over dinner at our apartment. "What a mess. And apparently the pandemic control group of the National Security Council was disbanded back in 2018. How bad do you think this is going to get?" she asks. You can't take the journalist out of my mom, who was the executive editor of the *New York Times* from 2011 to 2014 and is now on a sabbatical from teaching at Harvard to help out with my kids while Rob is in Boston. She is forever glued to the news and reads everything.

"We just don't know," I tell her honestly. "But I can tell you that people at the hospital are getting scared. The protocols are still totally unclear. A lot of people are talking about leaving the city." There are murmurs at this point among those who have the luxury of owning a second home. People have been quietly stockpiling supplies to decamp to the Hudson Valley, Long Island, Connecticut, or pretty much anywhere else they can get to outside of the city.

Somehow the threat still feels vaguely unreal to me, though. The messaging from our hospital leadership remains unflinchingly optimistic and I want very much to trust them. We are getting emails reassuring us that personal protective equipment (PPE) stores will be replenished soon. I believe them. Yet, I'm also happy about the doomsday stockpile my neighbor Kay is building in the storage unit downstairs—just in case. I'm sitting at dinner, smiling at my kids, but imagining how I'd convert our apartment into a makeshift clinic if I had to—if the shit really hits the fan. It's like my mind is going in both directions at once, caught between unbridled fear and the certainty that everything is fine.

After we finish dinner it's time to give the kids a bath and put them to bed. Bath time is when we all get to unwind. The bathtub is full of brightly colored toys, and Jonah splashes happily with a plastic duck while Eloise makes a "potion" out of their baby shampoo in a whale-shaped cup. I kneel down at the edge of the tub and watch them play, taking deep satisfaction in their temporary cleanliness and the fact that they are completely oblivious to the contagion that looms.

After the bath, my mom takes Eloise and Jonah to the bedroom for stories and lullabies and I call Rob. "I think the kids should go with my parents if this gets really bad in the city," I tell him.

Rob is not alarmed in the way that I am but he agrees. "Yeah, it's probably safer," he says. His calmness reassures me.

"Have you had any positive patients yet?" I ask.

"Nope, so far, so good," Rob replies.

We decide that we'll make a final call next week, when the kids are on spring break, about whether they will go to Connecticut, where my parents live. They have a house with a big yard in a small town: there's more space to play in an environment that feels safer. This is a huge privilege and I feel incredibly lucky to have the option to send my kids to a house with loving grandparents and some outdoor space to play.

"Worst-case scenario, the kids will miss a few weeks of school," I say to my mom. And at that point I still believe it.

SUNDAY, MARCH 8

"Eloise! We have to get dressed! It's Sybil's birthday party!"

Her friend Sybil's party is our last social plan before spring break, and Eloise is dizzy with excitement. The parents at her nursery school go all out for birthdays, sometimes even hiring professional party planners. It is really something to behold: at a given four-year-old's party there can be face painting, food trucks, personalized goody bags and gifts, magicians, and Disney characters. I'm not going to lie: I enjoy some of these parties. There are drinks and food for the adults, and while it can be intimidating to spend time with the posh moms of Eloise's classmates, it can also be fun to get to know them better. There is always a great birthday cake, and I get to eat Eloise's leftovers because she only likes the frosting. But the level of privilege and indulgence that my children have come to find commonplace in Manhattan does feel ridiculous and wrong. One of the reasons we've decided to move back to Boston is in the hope of finding a simpler and less extravagant environment in which to raise our kids.

I suppress my worry about whether it's safe to bring Eloise around so many other children and adults. There's a hushed sense of secrecy around the adult ICU at the hospital. We got an email from the hospital administration telling us about the first adult patients that were being admitted to the ICU with coronavirus a couple of days *after* learning about it on the news, which has eroded my trust and confidence in their leadership. We've been given very few details about the potential risk of transmission, and the communication continues to be limited. There's no clear timing on their plans to replenish our PPE, which continues to dwindle. Worst of all, there's no real data to help us understand the risks. I have a tendency to clench my jaw when I'm anxious, and the last few mornings I have woken up with a horrible headache from doing it in my sleep.

I've worked around contagious diseases my entire career, but until this point I've always felt that I was supplied with solid information and protective equipment to keep myself safe. I would feel so much better if there was some actual expertise or guidance on the risk of catching Covid while working at the hospital . . . but no one seems to have the answers.

The Princess cruise ship fiasco outside of San Francisco has solidified the sense that the coronavirus is quickly closing in on us from all shores. That's been underscored by the outbreak the first weekend in March just a few miles away, in New Rochelle, New

York, which is where Jane lives. But at his recent briefing Governor Cuomo said: "The facts do not merit the level of anxiety we are seeing." I've now lost a grip on what level of anxiety is actually warranted. My surgical training has taught me that panic doesn't serve anyone, and yet I can't help but wonder if that's exactly what I should be doing.

Eloise breaks through my silent worrying, and it's a relief. "I'm *so* excited, Mommy. I hope I get a goody bag." Her unbridled enthusiasm and zest for life grounds me. Today is a day of prioritizing her: not work, and not my persistent fears. This is one of the rare opportunities for me to just be a mom, and I am going to relish it. Today I'm not thinking about the things I encounter at work: a childhood cancer patient, or a baby born with a giant hole in her heart, or a mother who struggled for years to get pregnant and then after eight rounds of IVF went into labor at twenty-three weeks to deliver a child that fits entirely in the palm of my hand. We head outside and hail a cab.

When we arrive at the party, a pack of gorgeous moms descends on me. I'm always a little intimidated by these downtown preschool moms. They're impeccably dressed in designer jeans, thick cashmere sweaters, and perfectly beach-waved hair down to their waists. Their wrists are adorned in stacks of bracelets and their fingers showcase big diamond rings. It seems like an unspoken pact that to roll with this crowd you must have an impossibly slim body and undetectable Botox and fillers to disguise any hint of aging. Despite the fact that most of them have had two or three children, they look like twenty-three-year-old Pilates teachers. If I'm being honest, the geeky middle schooler in me has always longed for the acceptance of these kinds of women. But I tend to feel like a frump in their company.

Almost instantly, Erin, Arielle, and Samantha—three of the chicest moms at school—are peppering me with questions: "What's it like in the hospital?" "Do you think it's safe to be here?" "How bad is this going to get?" "Is New York going to be like China?"

The anxiety level in this crowd of parents creates an almost tangible buzzing frequency in the room.

"So far it looks like this is mainly a problem for the elderly, but, yeah, I think it could get bad here in New York," I answer, trying to be both reassuring and truthful.

"We're leaving for Southampton right after this. I canceled our ski trip to Colorado," Erin says.

Arielle nods in affirmation. "We're going to Palm Beach and not sure when we're coming back."

"I don't blame you for wanting to leave," I tell them, hoping that I'm hiding the part of me that's envious. I know that I have to stay and work at the hospital, where there's already been talk about travel bans. As the only healthcare worker in the bunch, I feel alone. I wish Rob were here.

———

The birthday party is winding down but Eloise clearly doesn't want to leave. She grabs a cookie from the table and rejoins her friends and they fall into a circle dancing to the Kidz Bop version of "Shake It Off" by Taylor Swift. The other parents embrace as they say their goodbyes, unsure when they will see each other again.

"Best party ever!" Eloise squeals up at me after we say our own goodbyes and leave, with her towing her custom goody bag.

"I'm glad you had fun, sweetie," I reply, sensing that it could be the last birthday party she goes to for a very long time.

WEDNESDAY, MARCH 11

Shit has met the fan. Any doubts lingering in me about the seriousness of Covid are gone. March Madness takes on a whole new meaning as public gatherings of any kind—sports, schools, concerts—are being shut down in all parts of the country. Office buildings are closing and the National Guard has been sent in to set up a containment zone in New Rochelle, close to Jane's home. At the hospital, the leadership has set up a Covid task force and has finally improved their communication. Each day begins with a briefing about the latest guidelines for testing and quarantine timelines after exposures. Then, around lunchtime, a hospital administrator records a message meant to reassure us that they've got things under control.

While it's clear they're making good efforts, the protocols are changing so rapidly that the illusion of control is clearly just that. Underneath the thin veneer of the administrator's messages is a hospital staff that is barely holding panic at bay at the lack of direction, the dwindling stockpiles of PPE, and the alarming sense that a tidal wave of patients is headed for the doors of our emergency room.

I function the only way I know how, by showing up each morning at 5:00 a.m. to take care of patients. In my rare free moments, I look at Twitter and Facebook, where I have joined communities of doctors sharing protocols and knowledge about how to treat coronavirus patients. A physician mother shares a link to the new Johns Hopkins Coronavirus Resource Center, which has launched a case tracker. Doctors out of the West Coast share PDFs of their Covid-19 evaluation guides and ICU protocols. They are all different. The posts I am seeing from doctors in Italy are the most alarming. The hospitals in the northern part of the country look like a war zone. They are quickly running out of ventilators and turning all of their units into Covid ICUs. They've even started using something called helmet ventilation on patients; it looks like a giant hood worn by an astronaut or a 1950s deep-sea diver that drives up pressure in an effort to stent open airways and lungs and deliver more oxygen. There's talk of having a proning protocol, which means having teams of hospital staff that flip patients onto their stomachs to encourage different parts of their lungs to expand.

One particular part of the post catches my eye. "Use of ECMO seems to be rare. Most patients do well on conventional ventilator management. ECMO is NOT your problem. Having enough ventilators and staff is." Angie is still on ECMO, fighting for her life and nowhere near ready to come off circuit. It's a relief, if only a small one, to hear it's unlikely that we'll run out of ECMO circuits, meaning there won't be any question about whether Angie can stay on hers.

As I go to scrub into my first case of the day, a routine appendectomy, I can overhear two seasoned nurses whispering about Covid. "If things get bad, I am *so* out of here," Margie says to Ann, the nurse who runs the OR board and the flow of operations each day. "After thirty years of nursing, I am not going out strapped to a ventilator." It's clear that she's not alone. More and more staff are calling in absent at the hospital, either because they're sick or because they don't want to come in. Our pediatric ENT department seems to have disappeared overnight. When I walked into the hospital this morning, I even noticed the number of security guards had dwindled. Honestly, I don't blame any of them. Part of me wishes escaping to the hills was a choice I could make, but I can't bring myself to do it.

The messaging everywhere is to "flatten the curve" and stay at home, wash your hands, and avoid touching your face. The transmissibility of the virus makes it clear that almost everyone is going to be exposed at some point. Our best hope now is to keep the rate of hospitalizations low enough that our resources do not become completely overwhelmed. I remind myself of a recent post I read from a doctor mom in Boston: "We just have to remember that most people have mild symptoms and most people will recover. We just have to remember to breathe."

My appendectomy patient is being wheeled back to the OR. *Just remember to breathe,* I repeat silently to myself.

When I get home later that evening, I see Kay and her husband, Nathan, loading up their car with their kids. They are officially evacuating to New Jersey. A few minutes later, Kay breaks into tears as she approaches me to say goodbye outside of our apartments. "I'm so scared. Please tell me our kids are going to be okay," she begs.

"I make this personal promise to you: I will not let your children die from this disease," I assure her. I choke back a lump in my throat. "We'll be celebrating together at the beach by the Fourth of July." I have to believe what I'm telling her is true to fight back an overwhelming sense of doom. I give Kay a bear hug and she disappears into the elevator with a stroller full of supplies.

Kay leaving means I'll be totally alone on the floor of our building once the kids and my mom and Magic go to Connecticut tomorrow. Rob and I have decided to go through with the contingency plan. After everything I've put the kids through in the last few years, being paged away from bath time and birthday parties and soccer games to go care for other people's children, the thought of bringing this virus home to them is too terrible for me to bear. At my parents' house, I'll know that they're safe and not trapped in an apartment without access to fresh air and space to run around. Our nanny, Pam, is a true saint and has agreed to go to Connecticut with them to help my parents for the foreseeable future. She feels good about it for herself as well. Her brother is a nurse and has also agreed that getting out of the city seems like the wisest decision. Hopefully it will only be a few weeks, but we really don't know.

When I walk through the door to the apartment, Eloise and Jonah are on the couch with Pam, singing "I'm a Little Teapot" over and over. Well, Eloise is singing and Jonah is just cooing at the older sister he idolizes. When Eloise cries, "*Tip* me over and pour me *out*," she flops onto the couch cushions, sending Jonah into a fit of belly laughter. He can say a handful of words and phrases at twenty months but has been slow to talk. He looks over at me with a huge grin and says, "I-e!"—which is how he pronounces "Eloise."

"Hi, munchkins!" I smile and go to drop my takeout on the counter.

"Shooshi?" Jonah asks excitedly.

I'm very predictable. "Yup!" I say, and he toddles over to sit on my lap as I eat my go-to New York City weeknight meal. Jonah loves to pick the salmon and avocado out of the rolls and nibble at the sticky rice separately. I savor the warmth of his squishy little toddler body on my lap as I devour my dinner in minutes. I'm always starving by the time I get home. Usually I'm so tired that the thought of getting the kids to bed is almost too exhausting to bear. But tonight I'm going to be present. Tonight I am going to treasure the bargaining and negotiating from Eloise and the fussing from Jonah. I'm going to lock the scent of their baby shampoo into my nostrils and snuggle them each a bit longer.

After a warm bubble bath, I dress the kids in their pajamas. Eloise asks for five books tonight. I practically have them all memorized. *Olivia*, the story of a naughty pig, is a particular favorite. "You know, you really wear me out, but I love you anyway," Eloise and I say in unison at the end of the book. Then I put Jonah in his sleep sack and carry him to his crib, his pudgy little fingers clutching his brown puppy lovey. He curls up into the corner near his taxi blanket and I sing the kids their bedtime songs. "Twinkle, Twinkle, Little Star." The alphabet song. "You Are My Sunshine." I tuck Eloise into her daybed, which houses a menagerie of stuffed animals. There is blissfully little protesting from either of them.

"Mommy, will you rub my back?" Eloise asks.

"Of course, love," I say.

You'll never know, dear, how much I love you

Please don't take my sunshine away.

The painful irony of the last line is not lost on me as I contemplate sending my little sunshines away for who knows how long.

SUNDAY, MARCH 15

Today the chair of the department of surgery sends our team the first in what he tells us will become daily updates about the department's pandemic response and priorities. A stoic surgeon with militant command of our department, our chair does not mince words. He informs us that we are canceling elective surgeries.

> The decision to cancel surgery was based primarily on an alarming shortage of resources (primarily PPE) that are equally essential in the OR and in the front lines of the COVID-19 battle.

It's astounding: we don't have enough PPE to keep the operating rooms open and protect our staff in the emergency room and medical ICUs. This feels unreal.

He tries to end the email on an upbeat note:

Let me emphasize that we're not overwhelmed yet! It's a beautiful sunny day. We have our families and friends. No matter how many of us get infected, the vast majority will do well.

I haven't been outside in sunlight for days. How is that supposed to be reassuring? At least he is acknowledging the very real fact that many of us will get sick, but the words "No matter how many of us get infected" rattle around in my head.

When I get home, I sit down at my laptop. My mind is racing. I start composing an opinion essay that I call "The Sky Is Falling." I write it because I know that hospitals need help. We will not be able to handle a massive surge of patients on our own. I've worked in hospitals long enough to know that our systems are not that nimble. The dwindling stores of gloves and masks are alarming. So I'm writing a call to arms to mobilize my fellow New Yorkers in the mission to get protection into the hands of healthcare workers in the city's hospitals, emergency rooms, and urgent care centers.

I jot down the following lines:

The sky is falling. I'm not afraid to say it. A few weeks from now you may call me an alarmist; and I can live with that. Actually, I will keel over with happiness if I'm proven wrong. . . .

I say this not to panic anyone but to mobilize you. We need more equipment and we need it now. Specifically gloves,

masks, eye protection and more ventilators. We need our tech-
nology friends to be making and testing prototypes to rig the
ventilators that we do have to support more than one patient
at a time. We need our labs channeling all of their efforts into
combating this bug—that means vaccine research and antiviral
treatment research, quickly.

. . . We might be the exhausted masked face trying to resuscitate
you when you show up on the doorstep of our hospital. And
when you do, I promise not to panic. I'll use every ounce of my
expertise to keep you alive. Please, do the same for us.

I finish the column in less than two hours and send it to my
mother. She responds quickly and says she thinks it's powerful and
good enough for the *Times* to publish. She gives me the email of the
op-ed editor. I take it from there.

MONDAY, MARCH 16

The chair uses the language of battle in his update today.

> Today the discussion of "re-deployment" is intensifying. . . . The emergence of this challenge reminds us that we are all employed in the delivery of health care. Our health care systems are at war with a pandemic virus. If your customary weapons are idling (heart surgery, for me) you are expected to keep fighting with whatever weapons you're capable of working. This means it's conceivable the surgery faculty will be needed in the ICUs, as one example. It also means that no one is on R&R. If COVID-19 accelerates as it did in Italy, there will be no "behind the lines."

I know that I've been well trained for this moment, and I've written in my op-ed draft that I promise I won't panic, but I'm scared. I never imagined myself as a soldier at war. The thought of redeployment—being assigned to a different department or unit—is unsettling. Yet, I do what I know is right. I add my name and my applicable skills to the redeployment list and wait to see what happens.

I have several good friends who served in the military, many in medical missions on the front lines of Afghanistan and Iraq. Bravery and self-sacrifice seemed to be part of the fiber of their being. The year before I moved to New York for this fellowship, from 2017 to 2018, I was a chief resident in Boston with my friend Geoff, managing the call schedule together for ninety type-A surgical personalities. Geoff had served in the Air Force as a flight surgeon and was deployed to both Iraq and Afghanistan, where he flew into battle zones to evacuate casualties and perform lifesaving surgeries. He also assisted in the response to numerous mass-casualty events, including bombings of a CIA compound in Khost, Afghanistan, and the H1N1 outbreak in Afghanistan. When Geoff told me war stories, I would just stare at him in awe.

"That's amazing, I could never . . . ," I often said.

"But maybe you could if you had to," Geoff would say, and smile back.

One Friday, when we were at the bar we often went to after a long week on call, Geoff told me a story that I'll never forget.

"We were on a mission in Iraq in 2008. I was on a helicopter with a group of Navy SEALs and they had a person of interest. Somebody had been helping to organize attacks on American forces, setting up improvised explosive devices. He was recruiting people to blow up Americans. The SEALs wanted to capture him to shut down the network. This was a typical mission and we flew close to where he was living. We landed a mile away from the target's house and the SEALs wanted to sneak up on him. We took off to refuel the helicopters. I was on board as the medical asset in case anyone was shot or blown up. When we were refueling, the SEALs were attacked and trapped in a firefight. They had probably been set up. We got a call early on the radio that a SEAL had been hit, so an emergency casualty evacuation was needed. We were spinning up the helicopter to go pick up the guy and we got a call that there was a drone overhead that had picked up our cell phone call. An Al Qaeda commander could be getting ready to give the command to strike down our helicopter with a missile.

"For a minute, there was total silence in the helicopter. Then I heard over the intercom: 'Doc, this is Pilot. What do you think?'

"'Well, we have to get our guy,' I answered him. 'This is why I'm here.'

"We flew in and the Al Qaeda operatives did try to launch an air missile, but the targeting system didn't work. This allowed our pilot to bank hard away from the missile and it missed us—just barely.

"It was a very sobering night, knowing there's someone waiting to blow you out of the sky," Geoff concluded.

I'm thinking back on Geoff's story. He had told me that he was terrified at the thought he could die that night but said he had felt certain in his choice: it was what he had signed up for. My situation now feels very different. Was risking my own life really what I signed up for when I decided to become a surgeon? No, it was not. Neither I nor any of my other colleagues outside of those with military experience or training in international aid work in conflict zones planned for anything like a pandemic. But it doesn't matter. It's becoming very clear that we're in the midst of something unique and catastrophic, the health crisis of a lifetime. I have to start thinking more like Geoff. Showing up to work is *my* mission now.

I hear back from the *New York Times* op-ed editor. There's no question: my mom's former position at the paper helps my submission get special attention from an editor who is usually deluged by submissions. Nonetheless, I'm thrilled to hear that the opinion section wants to publish my piece as soon as possible. Likely tomorrow. I run it by my boss for his stamp of approval and he warns me, "This is going to get a lot of media attention. And the hospital might not be happy about it." I nod in understanding. I know that I am taking a risk by sounding the alarm. The very title makes me feel like I'll be blasted as a hysterical Chicken Little, trying to scare the masses about the Armageddon. So be it. We're at war.

TUESDAY, MARCH 17

The column is published in the morning. I have no idea how many friends and colleagues will see the piece or what reaction they'll have. I fear the chair of pediatric surgery will be upset. I try to call Jane on my way to work but she is already distracted this morning with rescheduling one of her patients whose operation has been canceled.

As I walk into work, I can see that the emergency room is beginning to overflow. There are crowds of people in the lobby outside, lining up to be tested or treated for suspected Covid. We are already drastically understaffed. Anyone with even a sniffle has been sent home. I reread today's email from the surgery department chairman on my way up the stairs. In all capitals, in bright red boldface text, it says: "WE MUST PLAN FOR DEPLOYMENT ACROSS SERVICES."

All across New York City, those who have stayed—including my brothers and some close friends—are sheltering in place. Aside from "essential" workers like those at the hospitals, grocery stores, police departments, and transit systems, New Yorkers are sitting inside, waiting out what feels like an invisible storm. To many of my friends on social media, this seems to feel like a quaint exercise. People post pictures of cutesy homeschooling activities and baking projects. For many of those lucky enough to shelter in place, the reality and scope of the crisis have not yet registered. But I can see the alarming speed of this crisis both inside and outside the walls of the hospital.

In just the last forty-eight hours, they've built a huge testing lab right next to Jane's tiny office. Carts filled with tests are being wheeled into the lab by technicians in heavy PPE and nondescript white coats. I pass the lab on the way to my own office. I look over my list, which is unusually short. All elective surgeries have been canceled. But our urgent cases seem to have dried up as well. People are becoming scared to come to the hospital. I haven't taken out an appendix in over two days, which means there are children suffering with bellyaches at home. We usually see at least two to three appendicitis consults a day. The children's side is preparing to repurpose some units to take adults as needed. Instructions for rigging a single ventilator to accommodate four patients at once are being circulated on social media. The speed at which we shift from casual concern to full-blown disaster mode is just wild.

As I make my way to rounds in the NICU, one of the only places where we still have a good number of patients, I notice dozens of empty boxes that used to contain gloves. I resort to using a comically oversized pair just to examine one patient's wound.

"Have these been restocked at all in the last few days?" I ask the nurse at the bedside.

"Nope!" she says with eyebrows raised high.

"Well, that's not good," I mumble.

I continue on my rounds but finish early. With no surgeries to do, I walk over the skybridge to the Starbucks on the adult side of the hospital. I run into my friend Jake, who tells me the adult operating rooms are being converted into Covid ICUs.

"Just like Italy," he says.

When I get back to my desk, I tuck the N95 I used two weeks ago right next to my wallet in my desk. This mask is now my most important possession after my phone. When I need a new one, I'll have to get permission and then have a nurse get it from where it's kept under lock and key.

I open my computer to find that my op-ed has gone viral. I have a flood of media invitations. I don't have time to see a lot of what's been on television lately, but I've seen enough to know there are a lot of so-called experts peddling opinion, not science. The truth is we still don't know much about who will get the virus. Most of the Covid patients my hospital is seeing are the elderly, people of color, and people from systematically impoverished neighborhoods, but that's also our normal patient population.

On Instagram I have a lot of messages congratulating me on

the op-ed, but I also scroll past posts of my friends hanging inside with their kids at home, sharing memes and making jokes with the hashtag #socialdistancing. I am overcome by the sense that most people just don't get it. Outside of the healthcare system, why would they? I feel mounting rage nonetheless. Many people are still living as if this crisis isn't happening, and our healthcare system is not at all prepared to handle a pandemic. I try to channel my emotions into something constructive.

I accept a slot on CNN from host Don Lemon to appear on his show tonight virtually. I get home and find the one clean solid-colored top I have in my closet—I haven't done laundry in weeks—and decide to wear sweatpants, since no one will see my bottom half anyhow. I put on some concealer but don't have the energy to do any real hair or makeup; it would be inauthentic to even try to look put together. I have no gear or lighting to make my apartment look professional but decide the plain white wall behind my couch will have to do. I sit down and try to get comfortable with my laptop as I prepare to go live on TV. I log in to the show's guest platform via Skype and my heart starts to race. The show team greets me as "Dr. Griggs." Don's questions are smart, though mostly focused on conveying how terrifying the situation at the hospital is becoming. The segment is over in a heartbeat. I'm glad to have done it if it helps others take the pandemic situation more seriously.

WEDNESDAY, MARCH 18

Our daily update from the chair of the department reads:

> Our hospitals and our region are still in the terrifying, accelerating phase of new COVID-19 cases. The shortage of PPE continues to be critical. The PPE shortage may improve in the next few weeks, but not anytime soon. The ED is under serious pressure. Five Department of Surgery faculty have volunteered to be redeployed to the front lines in the ED. Details are being worked out as I write this. We should all be proud of their altruism.

Altruism or death wish? I immediately feel guilty for my cowardice. I signed up myself for the redeployment list, after all, but I'm not reassigned. Because, as a senior fellow, I am still technically a trainee, and I'm in a very specialized service, I have the luxury of some protection from redeployment. I have to admit, I'm relieved.

The emergency department is getting absolutely pummeled. "Right as I arrived, I walked straight into another intubation," my friend in the ED tells me. (Intubation means placing an emergency breathing tube through a patient's nose or mouth and down into their trachea.) "That has become the new norm." With staff testing positive each day, it seems to me to only be a matter of time before Jane and others get redeployed to the adult ICU.

My kids have been in Connecticut for almost a week, and I'm starting to get really lonely when I'm in the apartment. Rob and I FaceTime almost every night, but the sense of isolation is getting to me. "You should come stay with us in New Rochelle," Jane offers.

I accept. The idea of living in a house with Jane and her husband and kids is comforting—and probably low-risk from an exposure standpoint. Plus, we can commute together, which will be an easy drive now that there are so few cars on the road. I pack a suitcase and head to her house after work. We open a bottle of red wine and tuck into a wheel of cheese and try to think of a good movie to watch on Netflix. It's shaping up to feel like a bit of normalcy and a nice break, when Jane gets a call from her daughter's school.

"There's been an exposure and someone in Maya's class just tested positive," she tells me after hanging up.

Shit. If we both end up exposed or on quarantine, it will be a major problem for our department. Maybe it wasn't such a good idea to come here after all. "I better head back to the city," I say.

Jane just nods. This is a mess. I can tell she's worried about me as I head back out the door.

"I'm going to be fine," I reassure her, and hop into an Uber. As we whisk down the West Side Highway, I realize there's truly no sanctuary from the virus anymore. I feel ridiculous for increasing my exposure risk by traveling back and forth to Westchester in the same day. It's time to virus-proof my apartment as best I can and resign myself to isolation. When I get back to the city, although it's getting late, I feel restless. I head to Target to stock up on what's left of the cleaning supplies (everything with bleach is sold out) and canned soup. I scrub down every surface in the apartment with a water-and-vinegar solution and stock my little pantry. I unpack my suitcase and crawl into bed. My mom sends a picture of the kids tucked safely into their beds in Connecticut. "Thinking of you," she writes. My heart aches for them. I miss the sound of Jonah tossing in his crib in the next room. I miss finding remnants of Eloise's scribbled drawings and paintings on the counter. I even miss picking up the tiny loose socks and toys strewn around the apartment. There's no satisfaction in it being more clean than it has ever been.

FRIDAY, MARCH 20

The chairman's email tells us that the hospital has about 300 Covid-19-positive inpatients, with 200 more patients awaiting test results. That is almost a 50 percent increase in one day. There is also growing alarm about blood bank shortages because all blood drives have been essentially shut down.

Projections presented at noon today estimate that we will reach peak COVID-19 volume within 22-32 days, at which point the . . . system will need 700-934 ICU beds. The lower estimate exceeds our ICU capacity, even with surge construction, and [percent redacted] capacity added. With that resource limitation in mind, we have reduced the urgent OR schedule even more dramatically. . . . PPE is an increasingly limited resource, most dramatically illustrated by masks. N95 masks are already extremely scarce.

On a typical day, we are told, the hospital uses 4,000 non-N95 masks. Medicine, and especially surgery, is not a very environmentally friendly business. Right now we are consuming 40,000 surgical masks per day, and we are estimated to reach 70,000 per day. The downstate New York region is using about 3 million masks per week. "The entire United States strategic reserve holds only 75 million masks," the chairman's email warns.

I don't like that math.

The email concludes with the following:

The next month or two is a horror to imagine if we're underestimating the threat. So what can we do? Load the sled, check the traces, feed Balto, and mush on. Our cargo must reach Nome. Remember that our families, friends, and neighbors are scared, idle, out of work, and feel impotent. Anyone working in health care still enjoys the rapture of action. It's a privilege! We mush on.

I know he's trying to be inspirational, but my skepticism creeps back in. The hospital leadership is being cagey about the number of ventilators we have available. I won't be much use to the sledding team if my own lungs turn to mush.

SATURDAY, MARCH 21

The R.E.M. song "It's the End of the World as We Know It (and I Feel Fine)" is trending, as are memes of shoppers who have turned buying toilet paper into a blood sport. Nonetheless, my mother reports from Connecticut that no one seems to be wearing a mask there yet. I warn her to stay as far away from strangers as possible. Bringing the kids to the grocery store is not an option. The town playgrounds are out of the question too.

The chair's email message this morning is dark:

In broad strokes, we know New York is the national epicenter of COVID-19 infection, with a 10-fold increase in cases in just one week. To think we could mimic Italy seemed risible a week ago. Not today . . . In the past few days it has also become obvious that the virus has breached our Department walls, and we can expect to hear about increasing numbers of infected Department colleagues. It should be no surprise if these infections appear in clusters associated with the care of infected patients. This underlines the importance of deploying providers strategically to minimize the chance of incapacitating all or most of one subspecialty because of illness and quarantine.

101 years ago Lenin said "There are decades where nothing happens, and there are weeks where decades happen." This has been one of those weeks! A more modern revolutionary (John Wooden) said "Failing to plan is planning to fail." That will not be us.

It's hard to see how the plan is working. Doctors are getting sick. I decide to go for a run in a face mask. If I can wear it all day in the operating room, it shouldn't be an issue while exercising. My friend Alex, who is a first-year attending as a cardiac surgeon at a premier cardiac center out west, texts me while I'm jogging along the Hudson River: "My results came back positive for Covid." I call him; he sounds awful, with shaking chills and a fever that doesn't seem to break. "I'm scared, Cornelia," he whimpers into the phone.

Alex is my first friend to actually test positive, although dozens of people I know outside of the healthcare world have called with suspect respiratory symptoms. With few testing options available for people who aren't working in hospitals, there's little I can offer except to tell them to call me back if they have trouble breathing.

Alex sounds truly panicked, which is completely uncharacteristic. I've never seen him scared of anything. We met in 2010 on the same medical interview trail where I met my husband. We immediately bonded over our mutual love for New York and wise-ass sarcasm. The other applicants applying for the top residency spots seemed robotic. We became fast friends and decided to travel together after match day, which is the day when graduating medical students all across the country get their assignments for residency—or don't get one. We both got our top picks. Over the course of six weeks, Alex and I went skydiving and glacier hiking in New Zealand and scuba diving in Australia, rode motorbikes through the streets of Hanoi, hiked the temples of Angkor Wat, and danced until dawn at the Full Moon Party in Thailand. We had no idea how much work was ahead of us in surgical residency.

Alex tells me he is struggling to get out of bed. "I barely have enough stamina to walk to the bathroom." Then it gets worse. "Ally has it, too, and she's twenty-five weeks pregnant."

This is shocking news. Alex has always insisted that he doesn't want children. He and his girlfriend, Ally, are in great physical shape. They regularly post pictures of their glamorous lifestyle and luxury international travel on Instagram. They're "burners": utterly devoted to the annual Burning Man gathering at Black Rock City. I'm not sure whether to congratulate him or not. And I don't ask how he and Ally got Covid: whether they failed to act responsibly, in my estimation. Now certainly isn't the time to judge—not with both of them scared for their lives.

"That's terrifying, Alex. I'm so, so sorry," I offer, pathetically.

When I call to check on Alex again later that afternoon, he is driving Ally to the emergency room because she is having trouble breathing. I learn later in the day that pregnant women can no longer have a partner present for labor and childbirth in the hospital. The hospitals have decided that the testing shortage is too great and the risk to staff is unacceptable. While I support mitigating risk wherever possible, this move seems so dire. I would have been utterly devastated to deliver my children without any support by my side. Covid is polluting every aspect of our lives.

The day ends on a dark note with a direct message from a random person on Twitter. "So what if your kids get orphaned? That's why you and your husband get paid decent. Now shut up and do your job!" The profile photo shows an overweight, middle-aged white man in a navy suit, blue shirt, and red tie. This is the new American way: bullying strangers on social media. While social media feels like an essential lifeline to the outside world these days, sometimes acerbic messages like these reveal the dark underside of the ecosystem, and the dangers of making yourself vulnerable to attacks from strangers.

I think it's time to close my DMs for a while.

MONDAY, MARCH 23

The department chairman's emails are starting to go viral on social media. It turns out they provide some sense of comfort and reassurance to those outside our walls. Our hospital has started to trial the rarely used technique of ventilator splitting—putting more than one patient on the same ventilator machine—to conserve precious resources. I studied the technique earlier this month, when the possibility we would actually need to do this in the hospital seemed remote. But now it's reality. Today's email again encourages us to find inspiration in the chaos of it all.

The history of health care shows that wars are times of rapid acceleration in the art and science of surgery. Surgery takes the lead in many natural disasters. But we depend on others to lead us through plagues and epidemics, when it's our turn to fill whatever supportive roles are available, and cheer them on.

As one hand washes the other, today a technique forged in the crucible of mass trauma is helping our medical colleagues manage COVID-19. Turn, turn, turn! No one of us is smarter than all of us.

The use of a split-ventilator system (one ventilator for two or more patients) is a necessity. Equipment shortages have indeed become the mother of invention—or desperation, depending on your viewpoint. Today I decide to embrace this inventive attitude and build an N95 mask by attaching a filter to one of our plastic induction masks from the OR. I sit at my desk and watch a YouTube video with the instructions and briefly I am optimistic that I have found a clean and viable solution to the N95 shortage. But when I show the OR director what I've built, he informs me that the filter attachments are just as scarce as the N95s themselves, so it won't be much help. I turn my filthy week-old duckbill mask over in my hands at my desk. Once crisp, it's now wrinkled, and the previously white filter looks a little gray. The fabric is fuzzed out and the blue elastic on the back is losing its stretch.

My depressing trance is broken when my phone buzzes in the front pocket of my scrub top. It's a text from Kay.

"Hey."

"What's up?" I write back.

"Can you talk to Nathan? He is having shortness of breath."

"Of course. Call me."

Nathan walks me through his symptoms. He's not sure if it's anxiety or shortness of breath. He doesn't have a fever or any congestion. We settle on the fact it's probably not Covid. More likely he's having a mini panic attack—which, at the moment, is the better option. Kay gets on the phone. She tells me that Nathan's parents need them to move out of the house in New Jersey: it's too much with all the kids and the mess, and everyone is starting to lose their minds. "I'm pretty sure we are moving after this," she tells me. "I can't imagine being in the city all cooped up. This has been quite the eye opener. Anyhow, thanks for helping Nathan."

"Anytime," I respond.

"We're so proud of you. Love you," Kay adds.

"Love you too."

It feels good to be helpful to my friends, but I don't actually feel I have much to be proud of. I want desperately to escape from New York and get out of this mess. I long to be with my kids even if it means being driven to the brink of insanity from the lockdown. Though I can hear how maddening the circumstances have been for Kay and Nathan with her in-laws, I'm also jealous of the family time that's baked into their social isolation. My one luxury is that I have adult company and conversation every day, but I don't feel a compelling sense of purpose in being at the hospital right now. I miss my kids so much, I fantasize about quitting and walking away from all of this. I'm sure I could figure out something else to do with my life. I'm terrified that a prolonged separation could have a lasting impact on Eloise's and Jonah's development. Eloise should be in school, learning her letters and playing with crafts. Jonah should be in his little toddler gym and music class, learning to socialize. At the very least, I should be there to protect them and steer them through this scary and uncertain time in our lives.

What if this drags on and my kids are permanently screwed up as a result?

This fear of being responsible for some terrible outcome in my children's lives is nothing new. In fact, it's something that I've been dealing with from before the time Eloise was even born.

2015

In 2015, after Rob's initial cancer treatment, our lives briefly returned to a pattern of normalcy. We went on walks with our golden retriever, Magic. We were both in an "academic development" block of our residency, which meant that we got some time off from our hardest clinical rotations to do research. It was the perfect time to get pregnant, we decided, and we were lucky enough for it to happen.

Rob spent his days in a plastic surgery lab, building his research portfolio. I signed up for an elective in the pediatric burn unit. When we operate on burn patients who have lost significant skin coverage, we have to heat the operating rooms to sweltering temperatures. When I was four months pregnant, I found a storage closet with an ice vest and began wearing one every day in the operating room, taking quick breaks to replace the ice packs as they melted.

One night, I was paged to go examine a sick toddler with a fresh burn from a mug of spilled hot tea. Tears streaming down his cheeks, he was writhing in pain and had lost his IV in all the commotion. He was sputtering and coughing and the nurses were distressed because they couldn't get another IV back in. When a child has a big fresh burn, hydration is essential. The nurses desperately needed me to get a new IV in. "Hand me a start kit, please," I asked. His mother had left him at the hospital to tend to her other children at home. The nurses calmed the baby and I quickly and gently grasped his right foot. I slid the angiocath into his vein and snapped the needle back to reveal fresh dark blood, the sign that I was in. We hooked up the IV tubing and taped the IV securely in place. Success. It was a small win, just an IV, but it won me the respect of the entire nursing staff.

Little did I know that the toddler, in addition to his small burn, had a respiratory infection called parvovirus. Parvo is a pretty common infection in young children, who can infect the adults around them before they even start showing symptoms. In kids, parvo just means a head cold and a rash. In pregnant women, however, it can be a huge problem.

The next week I had a terrible head cold, but I was able

CORNELIA GRIGGS

to muddle through with Tylenol and extra fluids. When my fever broke, I developed a fine rash over my body. I called my obstetrician, but because I was seventeen weeks pregnant, they told me to just go and see my primary care physician. There wasn't much else to do. Embarrassingly, I didn't actually have a primary care physician in Boston—they say doctors are the worst patients for a reason—so Rob and I went to the hospital's same-day clinic on the advice of our friends in the medicine program. The doctor I saw told me it was likely a viral exanthem and nothing to worry about. That's a fancy way of saying I just had a normal viral rash and everything would be fine. She tested me for flu and strep, both negative. I was sent home reassured.

As I would later find out, I had parvovirus B19. Human parvo is one of the TORCH infections, a notorious group that are passed from mother to child at some time during pregnancy or childbirth. These infections can cause major congenital anomalies in affected pregnancies. I've taken care of these children many times. Some children get away with minor hearing loss and learning disabilities. Others have horrible brain damage to the point that they live their entire lives in wheelchairs and at special facilities for sick children. Many of them never speak or even recognize their parents. Another thing parvovirus can do in pregnancy is cause the fetus to have severe anemia. Some fetuses even

86

develop a deadly condition called hydrops, in which fluid builds up around the baby's heart, brain, and other organs.

About two weeks after I recovered from my cold, Rob and I walked to the hospital hand in hand for our anatomy scan, the ultrasound performed around twenty weeks of pregnancy that looks at the structure of the baby's organs. My pregnancy, other than severe morning sickness and that one cold, had so far been uneventful. We did all the normal early screening and even had the baby's chromosomes checked, just to be safe. After Rob's diagnosis, no amount of screening, testing, and reassurance seemed too much for us.

As the ultrasound technologist began the exam, we emphasized that we did not want to know the gender. Rob and I had both agreed that life has so few happy surprises left, we wanted that cinematic moment at our baby's birth announcing the sex. The tech squirted the warm ultrasound goo all over my belly and Rob and I giggled together with excitement as she showed us a tiny little foot. The tech glided the ultrasound over the other side of my swollen belly. We waved at the baby as the tech passed over a pair of bony little hands. But then the tech lingered longer and longer over the baby's heart. She stopped making jokes, no longer cooing and pointing out the baby's features. The air in the room went dry and I felt my throat swell.

"Is everything all right?" I asked.

The tech was silent for a moment and then put down the ultrasound probe, her face expressionless. "I'm going to go get the doctor. Hold on one second," she responded curtly.

No. Shit. Not again.

"What the fuck?" Rob said to me as the tech closed the door behind her. We didn't have to be doctors to sense this was going to be bad news.

An obstetrician came into the room and began repeating the exam. Rob and I were silent. But he was squeezing my hand so hard that my ring was digging into my skin and causing my fingers to throb. I started crying silently and prayed to my guardian angels: *Please, please, do not take this baby away from us.*

Breaking the long silence, the obstetrician was grave and careful with her words. "The baby has a lot of fluid around its heart," the doctor explained. "There is also fluid in the bowel. We don't know what this means yet but we're going to have to do some more tests."

Rob and I both sobbed. Once again our world was crumbling inside the walls of our own training hospital.

The next few days were a blur of tests, including an amniocentesis to check for infections and reassess the baby's chromosomes. My titers and amniotic fluid came back sky-high for parvo. We met with dozens of specialists, but very few people could give us answers about what would happen next. Even at Massachusetts General Hospital (MGH) in Boston and other hospitals we consulted that deal with the most complex fetal infections, no one could reassure us or give an example of a baby that had survived severe fetal parvovirus with hydrops and had gone on to live a healthy life. We're Jewish, and we met with rabbis. We called everyone we knew who would give us advice. We cold-called a very nice neurologist in the Netherlands who had written one of the only papers we could find on the outcomes of severe fetal parvovirus and hydrops, but even he had only seen a few cases of healthy survivors from severe fetal parvovirus like ours. Many pregnancies like mine resulted in fetal loss.

After one visit with an infectious disease doctor, Rob left the visit cursing God. "Why are you doing this to me?" he sobbed.

I had to get ultrasounds every other day to follow the changes in the baby's heart. There was a chance the baby would need a blood transfusion through the umbilical cord, a risky and semi-experimental treatment that carried a high chance of miscarriage.

After our last specialist consultation in New York City, Rob and I took a walk around the boat basin in Central Park. We had to make a choice about terminating the pregnancy or moving forward with a potentially sick baby. We are both pro-choice, and the idea of caring for a sick child after Rob's cancer diagnosis seemed too much to bear. But I had also learned that we were capable of more strength than we ever imagined we would need.

"I'm a doctor and a scientist," I told Rob as we stopped at a bench in front of a group of laughing children. "But I'm also a mother now. And I don't know how or why I know this, but I can feel this baby's life force and I know that they are meant to be here. And I also know that we are going to be okay."

What I was saying was: I simply couldn't terminate the pregnancy. I had never previously imagined that I would intentionally bring a child into the world if that life would be one of certain suffering. But a deeper, intuitive, and primal instinct in me knew that I was meant to carry the baby that was growing and fighting inside of me. Like me and Rob on the other side of his cancer diagnosis, I could just feel that baby was fighting to be alive. Pushing aside the fear and anger and resentment that we felt over Rob's diagnosis was the hardest part of continuing that pregnancy. We had come to understand that happiness and any sense of normalcy could evaporate in an instant. But I was going to have that baby regardless. "Okay, then," Rob solemnly agreed.

Two weeks later, the fluid around the baby's heart had resolved. It felt like a miracle. It was also total whiplash. The high-risk maternal fetal medicine team went from wanting twice-weekly visits with me to essentially dismissing us. My case was no longer interesting, which was a good thing. I've learned boring is the best thing you can be as a patient.

We also accidentally found out it was a girl. I devoted the remainder of my pregnancy to distractions with work. I wrote papers, took extra shifts, and sometimes snuck off to the ICU supply room to secretly ultrasound my belly when my anxieties were getting to me. Every time I saw that little heart beating away inside of me, I heaved a giant sigh of relief.

Then, in early October 2015, I gave birth. Our daughter was perfect. We gave her a Hebrew name, Adira Liba, which means "mighty heart," and took her home with the blessings of the pediatricians. It felt like we had skirted death once again.

TUESDAY, MARCH 24

My brain feels foggy today and I am plagued by constant nausea. When I get home, I call Rob. "I don't know what's wrong with me today. I can't shake this nausea," I tell him.

"Are you pregnant?" he jokes.

"That's not funny," I snap back. I have an IUD in place and Rob is likely sterile from the chemo he took in 2016. But I suck in a quick breath, the worry planted.

"I'm going to take a shower," I say quickly, and hang up.

I find an expired pregnancy test in the back of our bathroom cabinet. I pee on the stick and wait. I walk to the kitchen to prepare my lentil soup. This is silly. The odds of me being pregnant are exceedingly unlikely. But I feel like I've lost touch with reality. I return to the back room three minutes later. The test is clearly negative. I text a picture of the negative test to Rob.

"You need to chill!" he responds.

This morning the hospital announced that no visitors, including partners, will be allowed in the hospital with women in labor. We still know very little about the ways Covid might affect pregnancies and children. Pregnant women overall tend to have reduced viral immunity, so they are a particularly vulnerable population. A woman I know from college, Irin Carmon, who is a journalist, published an article in *New York* magazine on March 18 about being pregnant in the pandemic. Women are beginning to panic at the idea of delivering in hospitals overrun by Covid and potentially being isolated from their partners. Irin wrote:

> On March 9—an eternity ago in virus time—Boober, the service I had used to find a doula, sent out an email suggesting that people prepare for an unexpected "birth in place," or that they "consider the possibility of planning a home birth, if you have a low-risk pregnancy," lest hospitals be overwhelmed or too dangerous to enter. It seemed like an overreaction ("doula industrial complex," responded a doctor friend), but I decided to look into it for a story.

I'd watched a lecture once in medical school just in case I ever had to deliver a baby in the back of a taxi or the subway. I've always enjoyed a little mental thrill from the idea of a heroic moment. The reality is that most of the time when someone calls out "Is there a doctor on the plane?" the moment feels much more stressful or mundane than valiant. But now with Covid peaking, there are pregnant women across the country scrambling to prepare for a home birth they likely otherwise would not want or prefer. Irin described how some of the mothers she interviewed had "begun assembling the parts on Amazon, including scissors intended for animal umbilical cords."

Grocery shopping seems dangerous right now, let alone childbirth. Ally, Alex's girlfriend, was thankfully discharged home from the hospital a day or two after getting admitted. And after more than three days of running high fevers that would not break with Tylenol, Alex started feeling better. But all does not seem well in their home.

"She knew I never wanted kids," Alex moaned when I got a chance to catch up with him a few days ago and hear more about what's been going on. "And I have no idea when I'm going to be able to go back to work." He was still testing positive for Covid. "This is an actual nightmare."

"I wouldn't stress about that now," I suggested. "Just focus on getting healthy." But he's not wrong. It *is* a nightmare.

A cardiac surgeon cooped up at home with too much time is a recipe for disaster, and the stress of it, added to the hard time Alex was having coming to grips with the idea of fatherhood, meant he and Ally were at each other's throats and bickering constantly. Alex was criticizing Ally over everything around the house, monitoring everything she ate or did. His lack of enthusiasm about the baby didn't win him any points with Ally, either, of course. My image of them as the most Instagrammable, over-the-moon-in-love-with-each-other couple I knew has gone up in smoke.

There is so much uncertainty; what once seemed preposterous is reality. I think about the naïve optimism I felt bringing my own children into the world. And just a few short weeks ago I was delusional enough to think that the good life was just around the corner for us in Boston. Now I feel idiotic that I didn't pay closer attention to what was happening in China. I smugly assumed we would be better prepared or somehow better equipped in the United States. The coronavirus blinded me the same way that parvovirus did in my pregnancy.

Now most of us are checking our temperature, self-monitoring for symptoms, and wondering: Will this be the day I contract Covid too? I've now used my N95 for two weeks straight. Never in my wildest dreams would I have imagined that a disposable mask, pre-pandemic, would become a coveted treasure. Like people who lived through the Great Depression and continue to save and reuse tinfoil, I will never look at an N95 the same way.

Doctors and nurses at the hospital are freaked. New York City is not just overwhelmed but headed toward imminent disaster. Our worst fears are coming true. My op-ed title was not hyperbolic. On the adult side of the hospital, you hear a code being called every thirty minutes or so and teams are running frantically to put breathing tubes in patients before they crash.

The chair's email update this morning adds another terrible worry to the pot. It's clear some doctors and nurses will need to be laid off in the ensuing financial crisis hospitals will face after Covid.

Admissions of new COVID+ [Covid positive] cases to our system have continued to increase ~10% per day. ~20% are in ICUs, and ~80% of ICU patients require ventilators. Consult a compound-interest calculator to get a sense of how quickly we are approaching infrastructure capacity limits. We are scheduling very urgent cases in 3 ORs each day, with 2 rooms for true emergencies. Operating at 10% of capacity has an economic impact on a Department of Surgery that should be obvious to all readers. You probably realize that hospitals depend disproportionately on revenue related to procedures, and revenue related to COVID care won't begin to compensate. That must be as that must be, until the pandemic ebbs. Your Department is doing what it can to preserve cash flow. Our goal is to carry everyone through to the ebb, but exactly how we will achieve that remains to be seen.

As a brand-new hire, Rob will probably be first on the chopping block if his hospital is forced to do layoffs. While part of me wants to urge him to be careful, knowing his health history, I also know that he is younger than most of the surgery department and must prove himself useful if we want to maintain our livelihood. In that regard, perhaps the perverse comfort is that tons of staff at our hospitals are already voluntarily resigning. Some people have stopped showing up to work.

The chair's update ends with a reminder that healthcare workers are the most precious resource we have right now.

> This all boils down to the fact that health care is the most people-intensive enterprise of humankind. Health care workers are the limiting reagent for everything we do. Even if supply-chain victories suddenly leave us luxuriating in technology like respirators and ECMO, none of that is even remotely automated. A forest of bamboo bends to the ground in a typhoon but rarely breaks. We are that forest and we must not break. *By* the people, for the people.

And yet, many of us at the hospital don't feel that sense of camaraderie from the leadership. Though the hospital is going through a lot of masks, much of that is due to the fact that people are stealing them to take home. Crazily enough, many people are still not wearing them while going about their normal business, walking around the wards. Certain admins are even shaming some of us for wearing masks to protect ourselves. They say we are scaring the patients.

"I've never felt less like a doctor," my friend Meredith says with a sigh. She describes an experience with an administrator who warned her, "You'll create a panic wearing that N95 mask." My friend Amy, who is a nurse and six months pregnant, tells a similar story. "Our charge nurse looked heartbroken when she assigned me to a Covid-positive room," she said, "but all she could offer was one flimsy surgical mask."

A list of which procedures do and do not require N95 respirators is being circulated, supposedly based on CDC guidance. Intubation: yes. Routine in-line suctioning: no. CPAP: yes. Face mask oxygen: no. I can't make sense of these guidelines, and the distinction between the perceived safety of each procedure seems somewhat random. The guidelines are published without any apparent science as backup. If placing a breathing tube in a Covid-positive patient requires an N95, how is it safe to do deep suctioning of the same patient without the protection of one?

We are all suspicious of the narrative from administration: Are we being told we don't need N95 masks routinely because they don't have enough or because they truly believe they're not necessary? And if the wards and halls are safe without masks, why are all the administrators working from home?

A rapid-response team of surgical residents calling themselves the "SWAT"— the surgical workforce access team—is being formed to help with procedures across the hospital. The goal is to have the team expedite the care of Covid patients by taking over some of the procedures required and therefore easing the burden on the ER and ICU staff coping with the onslaught of Covid patients. Jane and the other pediatric surgery attendings who have not yet been redeployed have all volunteered for SWAT shifts. It's a remarkable testimony to the camaraderie of the moment. Surgeons don't do well with idle hands.

I tell my program director that I want to volunteer myself for SWAT shifts—as a pediatric surgeon, I'm good at putting in lines, so I can be useful—but he insists that I am needed in my current role as the pediatric surgery fellow. Many New York hospitals are closing their pediatric units and funneling patients to our hospital. I am not an attending yet and don't question him, but I can't make much sense of it. I think there is some fear that if I get redeployed, I will not be able to meet the requirements to graduate as a pediatric surgery fellow. There is no precedent for this scale of medical crisis to guide our training standards and requirements from the board of surgery.

WEDNESDAY, MARCH 25

The chair's email update begins with more of the same:

> It may be obvious that writing these updates is a daily struggle
> to balance terror with reassurance. Today the steady drumbeat
> of new cases continues, and it remains possible that our system
> will be overwhelmed. Repeating the threats represented by a
> lack of PPE and testing can feel corrosive. In sum, the acceler-
> ating pace of this contagion so easily overwhelms me that I risk
> becoming the Jaws of doomsurfing.

I feel that sense of doom at the hospital today. The testing
shortage remains critical. I want desperately to be swabbed to know
if I'm an asymptomatic carrier, but even my coworkers with fevers
or sore throats are being sent home without being tested. One

of our physician assistants, Kate, calls out sick with a fever. The hospital workforce safety and health hotline has been ringing off the hook and Kate says they tell her not to come to the emergency room unless she develops severe respiratory distress. In other words: *Too bad, good luck, come back only if you think you're dying.*

Yet, in spite of the PPE crisis and statistics showing that we are at increased risk of contracting Covid, my fellow pediatric surgeons and I continue to show up to care for our patients every day. The sheer bravery, consistency, and reliability of the remaining hospital staff is inspiring. As healthcare workers, many of us have a natural tendency to be "fixers" and problem-solvers: when we see a person in need, we run to them. But in the current Covid crisis, in doing so, we knowingly put our families and ourselves in danger. People start sharing macabre jokes around the hospital. Jane and I joke that we feel like Katniss Everdeen in *The Hunger Games*, volunteering as tribute. May the odds be ever in our favor.

I've become used to severe sleep deprivation and missing out on social events, holidays, even most of my children's early milestones. The altruistic part of my job is what I love most about my work. When a patient is coding—dying, to put it simply—in front of me, I never pause. I run to the bedside to do everything possible to save their life, especially when it's a child. At my hospital we specialize in something called ECPR (extracorporeal cardiopulmonary resuscitation), which involves putting a child on ECMO support at the same time the code team is performing chest compressions. Getting a giant catheter into a tiny baby's neck is challenging in any setting, but the precision required to get it right while the child is also receiving chest compressions—that is the hardest procedure I have to do in terms of technical skill. Still, our outcomes are impressively higher than one would expect. But the leaders of our ECMO team have called a meeting today. As a group, our ECMO team decides that ECPR is too dangerous in the case of a Covid-positive patient. The goal is to save net lives, and ECPR likely means exposing more healthcare workers and losing more lives on the off chance of saving a tenuous one. The pandemic means confronting ethically fraught balance tests like this one. The biggest one of all haunts me: What will happen if we run out of ventilators? If I get sick, will the hospital have one for me?

A former mentor of mine, a senior surgeon, sends me a text just as I am wrapping up at work. "Learn from my experiences here. I was in 9/11. Do the right thing for your family. My kids are petrified I will get sick and not come home. We have this sense as surgeons that we are invincible. As you're seeing we are not. You are senior enough not to have to be on the front lines. Be careful and protect your young family . . . Be safe my friend."

Reading this makes me feel like a terrible mother. My mentor is right. He is telling me to go home to my kids—to hold them and keep them safe as a devoted mother should. Ever fiber of me wants to listen to his advice and take the next train to Connecticut. What hubris has convinced me that I have any power to help these people in the hospital? The only thing I can control is my own little family. I have no idea how I will summon the resolve to show up to work again tomorrow.

THURSDAY, MARCH 26

Today one of the ER residents posts a video of the street in front of the emergency department, where there is a literal traffic jam of ambulances lining both sides of the road. The ER residents say their shifts are basically back-to-back "notifications," which are like flash flood warnings that go out to the entire ER staff when a very sick patient is arriving. One of them says the ER looks like a war zone, and he is former military, so it's not an exaggeration. They don't even have time to finish cleaning the rooms before they have to rush another patient in for intubation. Every bay is overflowing with sick patients coughing in masks—the haunting symphony of Covid. Plans are being made to park a refrigerated truck outside the hospital to serve as a temporary morgue.

Jane was already doing SWAT shifts, but now she has been fully redeployed to the adult Covid ICU. As a first-year attending— the lowest in the hierarchy of those who have finished their training—it didn't surprise anyone that she was among the first to be picked.

Though I have some protection from redeployment as a trainee, I still wonder if I'll soon be joining Jane in the adult ward. But when I ask my program director about it, he simply tells me, "We need you here on the children's side, where you belong." I do not question him, because I can see that our pediatric surgery service is still busy, as all of the hospitals in New York are sending their pediatric patients to us. The babies in the NICU did not, apparently, get the memo that this was a really terrible time to get sick. And so I get on with my work.

In addition to the severe pediatric emergencies, the children's side is filling up with Covid patients too. We've increased our age cutoff to help with the overflowing adult ICUs. I am taking care of young adults on ventilators, who seem to pop a new pneumothorax, or collapsed lung, every day. We even start seeing patients in their thirties and forties. So there's really no one spared from daily exposure in the hospital anymore. Still, there's no question the adult ICUs have it worse.

I go there during Jane's shift. She's rounding with a team of weary-looking residents. Their voices are muffled beneath their masks. With the constant beeping of drips and monitors and the deafeningly loud industrial fans and snaking silver tubes that have been set up for ventilation, they can barely hear each other.

Since my *New York Times* op-ed came out, people from all over the country have been mailing masks (including N95s) and gloves to my apartment. A mother from Iowa found me on Twitter and sent $1,000 worth of masks to me. Her husband runs a company that sells them. The simple kindness of these strangers reminds me why humanity is worth fighting for, even if it seems like there are so many people out there who refuse to do the right thing to protect themselves and others.

I arrive in the adult ICU in a mask, goggles, and scrub cap so no one can tell who I am and quickly and furtively deliver a fresh box of N95s to Jane's team. The masks haven't been approved by the hospital administrators and I would surely get in trouble if they knew, but going through the proper channels would waste precious time. No one responds to my emails to the hotline that has been set up for PPE requests anyway—they are all likely working too hard to address every email or tip that comes through. So I resort to being a masked vigilante.

The smile on Jane's face alone when I deliver the box is enough to make the risk worth it. I notice that she is not wearing any makeup, though—a huge deal for Jane. She always has perfect eye makeup on, even when she wakes up at 4:00 a.m. I've probably only seen Jane skip her morning makeup routine two other times before this, and those were both nights when she never left the hospital between calls. No makeup means Jane is incredibly worn down. It's only the beginning of her redeployment. I feel guilty leaving her in the ICU, but I have to get back to the children's side and my own patients.

On my way out, I can see for myself that what I've been hearing is true. The operating rooms have all been converted into makeshift ICUs. In each one there are two to four patients, all with Covid, hooked up to ventilators or anesthesia machines forcing oxygen into their devastated lungs. I decide that delivering masks will be my new secret mission. Like a fairy godmother, I will continue silently dropping them off to the parts of the hospital that are taking care of the largest numbers of Covid patients.

I feel particularly hopeless because Angie died today. Her lungs never recovered. She remained on ECMO for over a month, but then her other organs started to fail. When she died this afternoon, her mother's piercing wails filled the ICU. Our entire ECMO team was devastated. We almost never lose a child who was previously totally healthy, with no other comorbidities. ECMO almost always saves those children. Angie was in the same corner room in the ICU for so long, with pictures and decorations from her family all over. I will forever remember that room as "hers" even though I know hundreds of other sick children will pass in and out of it in the days and years to come. I go to scrub into a long abdominal case on a newborn, and then after I drop the baby off in the NICU, I become aware of a throbbing sensation on my face. I head back to my office, and when I finally peel the mask off, I can see in the mirror that it has left a deep groove over the bridge of my nose—a facial pressure ulcer from my mask. I look like I've been in a fistfight.

FRIDAY, MARCH 27

I'm stunned. Jane tells me that Dr. O., the senior surgeon who supervised the separation of the conjoined twins, is in the ICU with Covid pneumonia and it's so severe that he is on a ventilator. Apparently he's hovering between life and death. There are concerns that he may have caught the virus from a surgical patient a couple weeks ago—and that other team members from that case are now testing positive too. Superman is down for the count—this is a terrifying twist.

The grip that Covid has on our hospital feels suffocating. No one can think or talk about anything else.

I go to check on one of my young adult Covid patients. I am trying to protect my team both physically and emotionally, so I don't ask any of my junior residents to go into the room with me. I gown up and double mask, counting each breath. I take a look at the patient's chest tube and find that she is pouring out dark clotted blood into the canister. It's almost as if her lungs are slowly dissolving and oozing out day by day. With tubes sticking out of every side of her body, it's hard to recognize the person underneath it all.

And I can't shake the lingering worry that Angie might have had Covid. This patient is fitting a pattern we seem to be seeing with Covid patients. They are in a constant cycle of coagulopathy, bleeding and clotting, bleeding and clotting. It's something severe trauma patients do in a death spiral, and it's a very difficult cycle to manage. We give blood thinners in response to the clotting, then constantly need to stop them in response to the bleeding.

Next on my list is another young adult Covid patient on a ventilator. He is long and lanky, with a shaggy haircut. He's Dominican, like a lot of the patients in this neighborhood. But we haven't been able to locate his family, and as far as we can tell, he doesn't have any nearby. When I walk in the room, I can see that he has had a fitful day. The sheets are twisted and his body is drenched with sweat. I quickly confirm that all of his lines and tubes are working and in place. Part of me wants to linger in his room, to hold his hand and whisper words of encouragement. No one else is here to do it. But I wise up and decide against it. I need to be surgical. I get in and out of the room and on to the next Covid patient. *This damn mask better work.*

Around noon, the chair's email update hits my inbox:

The enemy is inside the wire. This became unavoidably obvious yesterday when another colleague was intubated. Just one of an unsettling number of new ventilator cases [here], but proof for everyone of how real this is getting, regardless of one's personal proximity to the razor wire and the Claymores. A widespread anxiety surge followed, with night-long text chains between the newly rattled. What is the proper response? First, at the most practical level, accept that there is no place to hide. The virus has no opinion on class, race, socioeconomic status, or professional stature. This latest reality-test reminds me that when I first bowed at the altar of healing, I felt I had cut a deal with the devil that I would freely sacrifice in countless ways for others, but in exchange for protection of my family. That lasted only until the first of several times that the devil reneged on our deal.

I know that raw deal all too well.

With more of our colleagues getting sick and being admitted to the hospital, the nagging reminder of our own mortality is undeniable. A common to-do list item now being discussed is creating or updating our last will and testaments. This weekend Rob and I updated ours. I utilize the free legal services from the hospital to get help with it. The lawyer who is assigned to me is eager to assist and thanks me for the work I'm doing in the hospital.

I imagine briefly where Eloise and Jonah would go if both of us died. Probably to my parents', but they're in their late sixties. I guess it's a conversation I need to have with my siblings. I have two brothers, Will and William. Will is my biological brother, and William is his best friend who lived with us on and off since grade school. Will and his wife are childless but are closest to our kids—the perfect doting aunt and uncle. But inheriting two toddlers would put a kink in their hip Brooklyn lifestyle. Will works in the music world and travels fairly regularly. Then again, Covid has already upended everyone's lifestyles. I resolve to have the conversation with Will and his wife. It feels morbid but necessary.

All over social media I am getting messages from friends: "Stay safe, we love you" and "Thank you for what you are doing." Some have even sent meals or extra masks to the hospital. My brothers, against my objections, have gone scouring every bodega in Brooklyn for extra N95s, gloves, and masks and drop them outside of my apartment door. "Thank you so much but stay home," I scold them via text message. On Facebook, my friend Hitha tags me in an emotional video of a new ritual where New Yorkers are clapping and banging pots and pans from their windows at the 7:00 p.m. shift change in honor of healthcare workers. I haven't heard it myself because I've been at the hospital so much. It makes me tear up.

For all the positive messaging being directed at me and other doctor friends, the appreciation represented by the clanging pots and pans is most deserved by the nurses, who are the real heroes of this disaster. Eighty-seven percent of the national nursing workforce is composed of people who identify as women, and if you stand outside of a hospital at 7:00 a.m. or 7:00 p.m. on a normal day, you'll see a flood of them sporting a rainbow of different-colored scrubs, wearing comfortable sneakers or clogs, toting lunch bags and large water bottles, coming from or going to work.

Adrienne is a friend and one of the best nurses I've ever worked with. Even as a seasoned ICU nurse, Adrienne has no control over her assignments. She has been pulled into a pop-up Covid ICU. For the first time in her career, she admits to me that she is completely overwhelmed. "I had two patients and I had two general care nurses with me," she tells me about her recent shift. "Both of my patients were Latinx women in their forties, both a little overweight, with mild diabetes. I felt overwhelmed by the anesthesia machines. I told the fellow working with me, 'I need you to gown up and show me how to work this.' So he did. The first patient had beautiful vital signs and then suddenly, while I was in the room, she coughed and vagaled." A vagal response—when the heart rate and blood pressure drop rapidly—is pretty common for patients with a breathing tube. A vasovagal syncope is also known as fainting. But for patients with severe Covid, even transient disturbances like a vagal response can send them into a tailspin.

Adrienne went on: "The woman's heart rate suddenly dropped from eighty to forty, so I quickly turned up the oxygen. But she was starting to crash. I was astonished. I have taken care of a lot of acute respiratory distress syndrome [lung failure] and pneumonia cases. 'Oh my God, she's gonna code just because she coughed,' I thought to myself. In that moment I felt extremely humbled. And I was blown away by how much the patients had in common. Everybody was the same. It was very overwhelming. I was looking at healthy forty-year-old women dying. It was the first time I felt my own mortality looking back at me."

The early epidemiological data from the CDC confirms that Covid can affect many age groups, not just the elderly. Among the hospitalized patients in some of the earliest cohorts, 20 percent were between the ages of twenty and forty-four. I haven't seen any data on race and ethnicity yet, but the early snapshot from our ICUs tells us that the majority of our hospitalized patients are Black and Latinx. This is an upsetting and cruel commentary on disparities and inequities in access to healthcare that existed well before the pandemic. Everyone may be vulnerable to Covid, but it's clear the systems that consistently marginalize Black and Latinx communities are working against their survival in the pandemic too.

Adrienne and the other ICU nurses have redoubled their efforts to communicate with patients' families even as many of them are reeling from Covid infections in their own homes and worrying about hospitalized loved ones.

"I've never had anxiety before, but I can't sleep," Adrienne tells me. "I am juggling my kid being homeschooled. But you can't phone it in in the ICU. You're either 100 percent present or you're gonna kill somebody. The pressure and stress are monstrous. Now I am not only taking care of my patients but I am guiding the other newer nurses. We are taking the brunt of it. We clean the rooms. We take out the trash and the linens. We are absolutely protecting anyone else from having the Covid exposure we are having. I don't want my nursing assistant who gets eleven dollars an hour to come in the room and get Covid."

The selflessness of nurses like Adrienne continues to astonish me. Her team has made a pact that no patients in their care will die alone. They are always in there to hold a patient's hand. They also never leave each other alone on a shift. "We went in for each other. That good old-fashioned nursing bond. Go a little bit more, a little bit harder, a little bit stronger," Adrienne says.

Even in normal times, what most people don't realize is that nurses are the ones who will make or break your hospital experience. When my mother was hospitalized for major trauma after being struck by a truck in Times Square in a hit-and-run, she had no recollection of the orthopedic surgeon who replaced her femur or the ICU doctor who tended to her drips while she recovered from massive hemorrhage. She remembers the kind nurse who stayed past the end of her shift to lift her out of bed and wash her hair for the first time. "Dance with me, baby," the nurse joked as she supported my mother in her arms. Another nurse gently tended to the bedsore she developed on her back, which was the most nagging and painful injury of all even after several crushed bones. The experience of anyone who has a long hospital stay is always marked by the caliber and care of the nursing staff.

That's why the nurses deserve the clanging pots and pans even more so than the doctors. I have so much admiration for Adrienne and the nurses here in New York. When we talk about the front line, nurses are shouldering most of the hardest work of this pandemic. Both at home and in the hospital, they are the glue holding it all together.

But how long can they keep going like this?

SATURDAY, MARCH 28

When Jane and I are paired together on call, our team often labels us with the gallows-humor medical phrase "black clouds." It always seems like the most life-threatening, complicated cases wait to roll into the hospital at those times.

Today, Jane and I are both on call in our regular pediatric surgery roles. But these aren't regular times. A baby at another hospital in an outer borough, already on a ventilator, is being rushed to our intensive care unit. His mother is also on a ventilator and is positive for Covid. The baby is not getting better on the ventilator. He needs ECMO to do the work that his damaged lungs no longer can.

This is the kind of case I've been dreading. We haven't seen many cases of Covid in infants. ECMO is extremely rare for a baby to require. Yet, inside our hospital, our days and nights are beginning to be filled with emergency cases like this one that none of us have ever seen before.

Jane and I get to the hospital and prepare for the case. When the infant arrives, he looks frail and tiny in his isolette, a clear-plastic–covered bassinet on wheels that we use to house critically ill newborns. His skin is already ashen gray, a sign of acute oxygen depletion. When a baby is struggling to breathe, you can see each tiny muscle in their chest fighting to gasp for more air. A blood gas test reveals critically low oxygen levels. He needs to go on ECMO quickly to have a chance at surviving.

Performing ECMO is like doing a swift, intricate dance. My job is to cannulate the baby's neck vessels. That means placing large catheters that will suck out the baby's blood to be passed through an oxygenator in the ECMO circuit, which filters out carbon dioxide and uses an oxygenator to send oxygen-rich blood back to the body through another large catheter. The perfusionists help prepare the ECMO machine and most of the supplies.

I cut the baby's neck open while Jane swiftly encircles the tiny blood vessels, and then we move in tandem from muscle memory. There are some tricky moments—the ECMO cannulas are being finicky—but in only thirty minutes we are finishing up. I hold the cannulas and tubing in place near the baby's head while Jane sutures it all down so nothing can move or be dislodged. The thick plastic tubing in my hands pulses with warm blood. The ECMO circuit is now infusing the baby's blood with a rushing river of oxygen and nutrients and giving his lungs a total rest. We did something good today.

But the sense of accomplishment can't fully mask my fear. When we put a patient on ECMO, there is usually a crowd of ten or more in the room, watching and helping. Today they are all huddled outside the room behind glass doors. In the past, I felt pride that I was one of just a handful of people in the hospital who could be at the table during ECMO; I was the one *doing* the cannulation instead of watching it behind a crowd on tippy-toes. But the price of being close to the action now is proximity to danger. Would it be possible for this baby to transmit Covid to me and Jane while intubated on ECMO? Unlikely, but no one really knows.

I peel off my gown and blood-stained gloves, drenched with sweat beneath the sterile garb. My entire body feels tense. We only have twenty or so ECMO circuits available for the whole hospital. We have hundreds of patients currently on ventilators and not improving. I think of Dr. O. Will there be a circuit for him if he needs it?

Jane turns and heads toward the empty operating rooms downstairs. I follow her, worried she's mad at me for struggling a bit with the cannulas. It turns out she wants to check her own oxygen saturation because she is suddenly overcome by the sensation of gasping for air. That is the kind of stress we are under. When her oxygen sat reads 100 percent, we both laugh at ourselves. The two of us go into Jane's airless office, not bigger than a supply closet. It has become our comfort station and we often gather here to regain our bearings.

This time we are both laughing and crying in a combination of relief and despair at how absurd the entire situation feels.

We healthcare workers are all overwhelmed, exhausted, and increasingly angry over the total lack of preparation and the life-threatening dearth of basic equipment. Inside our hidden comfort stations, away from the eyes of patients and often (in the case of women like Jane and me) our male colleagues, none of us are certain we have the stuff—the technical skill, stamina, and moral courage—that is so desperately needed. I don't know how long I can sustain the modicum of bravery I have left. Today I feel desperately that, if I had the option, I would just escape this place and quit. I want to hunker down in Connecticut with my kids. But if I do that, I won't be able to graduate. I'll be flushing away everything I've worked for over the past decade. And no one knows how long Covid will drag on. Weeks? Months? Years? If this is what medicine looks like for the rest of my career, there's no way I can sustain it for a lifetime. I'll figure out a way to do something else, even if it means giving up operating—which would break my heart. Still, staying alive—and sane—for my kids means more to me than anything else.

"Do you know I used to secretly use the ultrasound on myself to check Eloise's heartbeat when I was pregnant?" I tell Jane. "I was convinced she was going to die up until the very last day."

"Griggs, everybody does that." Jane laughs at me.

Something about having Jane tease me makes me feel a little less ridiculous.

———

After pulling myself together, I take a minute to check my phone. There's a bar graph on Twitter that haunts me. It shows the U.S. case numbers compared to Italy. We're a few weeks behind but facing the same merciless Everest-like curve of the rise of cases there. It seems like we have such a long way to go until we're through the worst of it.

Also on my phone is a text showing pictures of Eloise and Jonah. I haven't seen them in more than two weeks other than on FaceTime before they go to bed. In the photo their visages are covered with Day-Glo face paint lovingly applied by my mother. My mom and our close friend Marsha, who is isolating with my parents, are running a makeshift nursery school over Zoom in Connecticut. My mom is also teaching her Harvard students remotely. The kids are safe and being cared for. In this latest picture, they're enjoying a sunny weekend. I feel a sharp and probably selfish pang of self-pity at missing out on the fun and being locked in my depressing surroundings.

I need to vent. I start tapping out a tweet, because I want my friends and family to hear and see me. I barely have any followers anyhow.

"My babies are too young to read this now. And they'd barely recognize me in my gear," I type under a photo of myself that I took just before Jane and I started the ECMO procedure. I'm wearing a thin paper gown, a blue hairnet, and an N95 under a surgical mask. I have on my headlight and the magnifying glasses that are required for operating on tiny infants. I look unrecognizable under all the protective gear.

I add a third and final sentence to the tweet. "But if they lose me to Covid I want them to know Mommy tried really hard to do her job."

SUNDAY, MARCH 29

Oops. That tweet has gone completely viral.

Hospitals get very cagey when staff post anything work related on social media or speak to news outlets. Fellows are supposed to put their heads down and work, and posting on social media is often perceived as an attention grab. I feel a little embarrassed, wondering if I wasn't being very professional. But the greatest worry and top priority of hospitals is patient privacy and protection, which is hugely important to me, too, and there's no risk of me having run afoul of anything there. The photo didn't have any patients in it or identifying information.

I think about my responsibilities as well as my relationship to public media as I prepare for rounds. I have no intention or desire to become a hospital spokesperson for Covid, but I also know that I am in a unique position because I have already signed a new job contract and am just three months shy of graduating from my fellowship.

That makes getting fired for speaking out unlikely and protects me somewhat from the kind of scrutiny and punishment that younger residents or more senior, permanent staff might face. I know that many others feel silenced. I wrote the *Times* op-ed. Is there more I can do to tell the world about what I'm seeing in the hospital? Would it help?

I have some experience in media. In medical school, I worked for a year as a research assistant to Mehmet Oz on his television program, *The Dr. Oz Show*. At the time, Oz was still a widely revered cardiac surgeon at the hospital affiliated with my school. He had started his show after a couple of years of doing spots on *The Oprah Winfrey Show* that were medically sound. Sure, like many surgeons, Dr. Oz skewed conservative, but the opportunity to work on his program was a chance for me to flex the journalistic side of my brain. Overall he was a kind, good boss and supported my application to surgery residency. But there were also things about working there that ranged from the strange to the morally concerning. He would ask me questions on the spot like "What is the gestation period of a polar bear?" and expect me to come up with the answer right away. The demand to keep ratings high meant his producers often pressured me to vet medical advice that I felt was questionable at best. I felt a conflict of interest. When Oz got involved with the Trump administration, and what I believed to be his already-established habit of recommending treatments or cures with little to no evidence behind them seemed to me to be getting worse, I was disappointed.

It struck me as the sort of dangerous outcome that an obsession with celebrity can result in.

Nonetheless, as a result of working on the show, I understand how to package complex medical concepts into sound bites that resonate on TV. My mother's journalism contacts also mean that I have quick access to editors and reporters. And for what it's worth, I have long been a loudmouth, calling out injustice when I see it. During my residency in Boston, I sounded the alarm on unfair treatment of childbearing surgical residents and landed myself in the *Boston Globe* looking pregnant and pissed off in my white coat. So the hospital knows who they've hired.

I do think that everyone deserves to have a window into this tragedy. There are currently no reporters allowed inside our walls: it's considered too dangerous, given the uncertainty about the transmissibility of the virus. What if I were to become that reporter? There are still so many people across the country that don't believe this is real. They're calling it a hoax by the media. Maybe I can be a portal to our reality inside the hospital.

Right now, the truth for me is that Covid is fucking scary. I keep having moments of dissociation when I feel like I am watching myself in a movie. A psychologist would probably tell me that this is a response to trauma. No living doctor has seen anything quite like what we're living through. I don't care how seasoned you are—whether you're a Navy SEAL in combat or an ICU nurse with forty years of experience—absolutely no one is prepared to see this much suffering and death all at once. Every New York City healthcare worker of this generation will be forever haunted by this time. But in these dissociative moments I try to remember that I am living through a historical moment, and there has to be meaning in that. It's why I'm writing all of this down. Writing it all down is my way out and a way forward. It's the only way I can meaningfully process what I'm seeing and thinking and feeling. There will be time for therapy after this. If there is an after.

Lately I am ruminating on a quote from Albert Camus's *The Plague*. The French philosopher and author wrote the book after immersing himself in the history of the great plagues of history, such as the fourteenth-century Black Death that killed millions of people in Europe and the Great Plague of London from 1665 to 1666.

There is a character in the book named Dr. Bernard Rieux who works tirelessly against death and tries to lessen the suffering of those around him. "This whole thing is not about heroism. It's about decency," Camus writes. "It may seem a ridiculous idea, but the only way to fight the plague is with decency." A character asks Rieux what decency is. His response is as clipped as it is eloquent: "In general, I can't say, but in my case I know that it consists in doing my job."

This concept of decency is becoming my guiding light. I'm losing so much faith in our institutions of power: the federal government, the state, and now the very hospitals and healthcare systems that employ me. If there's one thing I want to live up to, it's maintaining human decency. And, like Dr. Rieux, the most decent thing I can do right now is my job.

But that doesn't mean I have to put my head down and shut up. The real heroes around me—the nurses, the environmental services team, and the patients clinging to life—deserve to be recognized, protected, and treated better. If this costs me some resentment from others who think I am not "front lines enough" to be speaking up, I can live with that. Hospital egotism is nothing new to me. It's true that I'm not on the front lines the way that the ED doctors and nurses, the ICU team, or the anesthesia and intubation teams are, but I've worked here for so many years now—in medical school, for my first two years of residency, and now as a fellow—that I have friends in every department. I'm able to weave in and out of all of these places and see what's happening.

There will always be someone who suffered more, who worked harder, who had it worse. But as one of my wisest friends told me: suffering is not a competition. Many of the older surgeons who trained me like to remind the residents how much harder things were in "their day." Decades ago, surgical trainees quite literally lived at the hospital during their training. It's why we are called "residents." But there were also parts of their lives that were simpler. They didn't have nearly as many administrative duties or as much paperwork to manage. There were fewer treatment options and therefore fewer medications to remember. Nurses often catered to the residents in the old patriarchal days of surgery—not that I wish for a return to that sexist system at all. And regardless, I can only know and speak from my own lived experience. I'm not going to let the resentment from others invalidate that. The way I see it, human connection and compassion is possibly the only way out of this giant tragedy. That's how I doctor and it's how I'm going to speak. I'm not a philosopher, but I know how to describe what I see so that people will know this is real, this is happening, and we can't afford to ignore or deny it.

The people I care about most are Jane, my chief, my program director, and the nurses. I know they will set me straight if I step out of line. And I will shut up if they tell me to. But when I head upstairs to start my rounds in the NICU, I am immediately stopped at the door by Sylvia, my favorite NICU nurse. She's heard about my tweet and my op-ed. "Thank you for doing what you're doing, Dr. Griggs. We are proud of you," she says, nodding.

Sylvia is an old-timer, a baby whisperer, and is often assigned to the sickest babies on the unit. She's trained generations of nurses here at our hospital, known to be one of the greatest nurseries in the world. The NICU nurses are a special club, and it takes time to earn their respect. Nursing the tiniest and most fragile newborns, some of them weighing less than a pound, is a true art form. The protocols, dosing, and management are entirely different from every other part of pediatrics and medicine. Pediatric surgeons revere the best NICU nurses and know not to piss them off by unraveling their perfect swaddles or disturbing a labile baby on their watch. Sylvia in particular is known for hazing the junior pediatric surgery fellow:

if you do a procedure poorly or even look at a baby the wrong way, she will rat you out to the chief without hesitation. Even if she's not on, her clique of nurses is always watching.

I spent months winning Sylvia over when I first started, greeting her at 5:00 a.m. with a smile even when I could barely keep my eyes open, knowing her opinion mattered. If Sylvia approves of my writing and posts, I'm going to be all right.

I think about how much good has come from speaking out already. After writing my op-ed, people sent in all those masks. I was able to mobilize a group of medical students who are now also accepting donations of PPE. Other people have contacted me to donate boxes of iPads and other gifts to the pediatric patients at the hospital currently stuck in isolation away from their parents.

I decide to accept another invite to appear on CNN. It's clear that a lot of people in the city still have no real grasp on what it looks like on the inside of our hospitals right now. After I finish the interview, I get a lot of responses that make me feel people are connecting to my message, particularly women. I think it's because, although the media and the public want to glamorize healthcare workers as heroes, the notion that we are also mothers, sisters, spouses, and daughters pulls on heartstrings.

MONDAY, MARCH 30

My mom sends me a video of the kids playing outside in her yard. They have constructed a makeshift terrarium in a cardboard box labeled "Coldie the Worm." Eloise gently cups the wiggly worm in her tiny hands and coos at him lovingly. Though it still seems that very few children are becoming severely ill with Covid, sometimes I worry they could be silent carriers, and I wonder if I've made a huge mistake and put my parents at risk. There are no easy decisions these days.

The video reminds me they are getting fresh air and playing in the yard. I wouldn't be able to give them any semblance of that here in the city. I know my parents, along with our nanny, Pam, and our friend Marsha, are doing their best to preserve some sense of normalcy.

"Please tell me you're being super careful," I write my mom.

"I promise, we are. I love you and I am proud of you," she writes back.

When I get home the *New Yorker* magazine is in my mailbox. The cover art shows a woman in a hospital, in full Covid gear, video chatting with her children and partner from her phone amid a chaotic scene of crashing patients being wheeled through a hallway packed with gurneys.

———

Kay texts me from New Jersey. "I hate to complain to you, but living with my in-laws is going to be the end of me," she writes.

"Oh, please complain. It's nice to talk about something besides the hospital," I reply.

She's not the only friend I've heard from who is finding that sheltering in place has a way of magnifying familial tensions. What once felt like a temporary, cozy experiment in indoor entertainment has now evolved into a prison for parents and especially mothers, many of whom are juggling the emotional weight of the Covid crisis, negotiating complicated family relationships, caring for multiple kids, figuring out what to cook, trying to work from home, and more.

Marsha, who runs her own small business as a children's occupational therapist, is basically running a home school for our kids in Connecticut while simultaneously figuring out how to convert her entire practice from in-person to online. Her clients are largely well-connected Manhattan families and they have high demands for their children. She also keeps everything running in her own family and is under incredible pressure to keep them all afloat right now. Marsha is particularly paranoid about catching Covid because she has asthma and is convinced it would be a death sentence for her. "I'm just saying this because I need to say it to someone," Marsha told me. "If I am intubated and sick with a poor prognosis, play recordings of Josephine's voice. I think it would bring me back." Josephine is her daughter and Eloise's best friend.

The speed and determination with which these women have transformed their lives is dazzling. It's true that my job involves physical risk of Covid exposure, but at least I get to leave the house and talk to other adults. At least there are brief moments of normalcy sprinkled into my work. I start to think that I would be going absolutely insane if I were stuck in the house with the kids, unable to perform my job or direct my nervous energy into something that felt like a productive contribution to the crisis. Maybe I am the lucky one.

Then my friend John, who normally lives in Florida, texts me a picture of himself in the PPE they've been supplied with on the USNS *Comfort*, a huge emergency relief ship that has just arrived in New York with military doctors and personnel on board to assist in medical disasters. They have full military-grade respirators to protect their staff. I don't know any doctor in New York who's been able to get ahold of that kind of high-quality PPE. They're sold out all over the globe, likely for months to come.

And suddenly I am furious again. John is a good guy and

genuinely believes he's here to help us out, but people who are outside of New York just don't get how bad it is. He doesn't realize how insensitive it is to show how great his protective gear is when I've been reusing the same flimsy N95s a minimum of ten times in Covid-positive rooms. Even after getting the donated masks, I need to make sure the supply stretches out as long as possible.

My anger is not really with John, though. It's with the federal government and the leaders of our healthcare systems. I am enraged that people predicted this pandemic months ago but it still feels like our leaders did nothing to proactively protect the talented and selfless people I work with at the hospital. As they say, denial is not a strategy. I am furious at the human cost in already vulnerable communities of the city, where so many essential workers have no choice but to risk their health for low-wage jobs in grocery stores, transportation, and other places. I am ashamed of who we are as a country. When I see images of Chinese doctors and nurses in full hazmat gear, I am reminded of our technological and manufacturing shortcomings.

I am furious at my own idiotic blindness, believing that our healthcare system was one of the best in the entire world, that we would be infallible and unscathed in comparison to countries with fewer resources. I studied health policy in college and medical school and am pretty well-versed in the general shortcomings of the U.S. healthcare system, including our archaic payment models, our pitiful access to primary and preventive care, our woeful racial and socioeconomic disparities in outcomes, the pathetic maternal and infant mortality rates, and the unfathomable expense of the entire system. At the same time, I always took some comfort in the idea of American exceptionalism in healthcare. Despite falling short on basic health metrics, we do have access to some of the most technologically innovative and surgically sophisticated systems in the world. That's part of what makes being a surgeon here so much fun. I've assisted in operations on fetuses in the womb and taken organs out of bodies with the help of a robot. I wrongly assumed that the awesome U.S. technological advantages would protect us from infectious disasters like Ebola. But that's because I was naïve and didn't truly understand the epidemiology of a contagion like this one. Few doctors did, even those in the highest positions of power in government.

When I traveled through Asia in 2011, I found the custom of wearing a face mask somewhat curious. Now I will never view an airport, a salad bar, or a packed concert hall with the same casual ease. In the medical field, you are discouraged from taking sick days unless you are practically on your deathbed. I cannot count the number of times I worked and operated through a terrible head cold. During my intern year, I even completed an entire twelve-hour shift while attached to an IV because I was so dehydrated from a bad case of food poisoning. My colleagues praised me for this "toughness." Surgery trainees were known to share a morbid joke in residency: "If you miss a day of work, we want to know your hospital room number and the ventilator settings."

In pediatric surgery, we have a joke that by the time you're done with fellowship your immune system is practically invincible to all the common viruses. A well-known phenomenon is to spend the first six months of your junior fellow year sick with a string of constant coughs and colds because we are exposed to so many sick children on a daily basis. It's part of the hazing period of our training. The peeling red pleather couch that has been in the fellow's office for over twenty years now has to be seen as a health hazard.

One of the worst days of my fellowship was spent largely on that couch, too weak to get myself home, struggling through a twenty-four-hour shift with the worst stomach cramps of my life, a throbbing headache, and uncontrollable vomiting. I took pages and gave orders from my cell phone and luckily made it through the night. When I finally stopped vomiting, I could barely stand. Most people would probably have gone to an emergency room, but doctors are the absolute worst patients, and in classic form I was determined to tough it out on my own. Now the idea of showing up to an office with a phlegmy cold, coughing and sneezing all over, sitting on that shared couch, is revolting. My new morning ritual is to bleach down my entire desk, including the keyboard and phone. The astringent, stinging sensation of bleach fumes in my nostrils is reassuring.

WEDNESDAY, APRIL 1

April Fools' Day starts with another overnight ECMO cannulation, but thankfully this one has nothing to do with Covid, just the more typical heart failure. Still, the child will take up a precious circuit. I never imagined that resource allocation would even enter the calculation in our decision to provide lifesaving treatment to a child. But in this case, her chances of survival are super slim at most. Did we make the best decision using a circuit for this child, on the rare chance that she would become eligible for a heart transplant? That was her only hope for survival. But the idea of putting a child on the heavy immunosuppression required to keep a transplanted organ alive is terrifying too, given the current climate. We warned the patient's mother about all of these risks, that the chances were slim. "Please, please do whatever you can to keep my baby alive," she pleaded. What parent, when faced with the life-or-death decision to save their baby's life in the middle of the night, would choose otherwise?

I'm allowing myself some hope today that resource allocation considerations will soon lessen. In March, Covid cases were doubling every three days in New York. Now the rate is slowing: they're doubling only every seven days.

The morning after the cannulation, I walk across the skybridge to Starbucks and find Erica, my favorite barista, working. She sees me in line and flashes her signature half smile, which means she's going to start preparing my regular cold-brew coffee order before I even get to the register. My conversations with Erica are a reliable bright spot in my day, and the hard-boiled eggs and cheddar protein box is my main source of nutrition. I've just about lived off of them since med school. When they recently started putting little everything-bagel seasoning packets inside, it was a total game changer for me.

"Helloooooo, Cornelia," Erica sings when I get to the front of the line.

"Helloooooo, Erica," I answer. "How in the world are you happy right now?" I laugh.

"Listen, I'm alive and I've got a job and that's what's good for today, all right?"

"If you say so," I reply.

"It's bad up there?"

"Children's side, not as terrible, but the adults, they're hit hard," I say.

"You got this," Erica says as she hands me my drink.

"Just keep bringing the caffeine and we will all get through," I say with a smile.

As I walk back across the skybridge nursing my cold brew, a hilarious text comes through from Marsha. Somehow Eloise and Josephine have gotten into a stash of old pasty sunscreen. They've caked their faces and hair in a goopy white slime while playing "salon" in the bedroom. The adults have just discovered the giant mess they've made. The video on my phone shows the girls giggling uncontrollably in a pile on the floor as Marsha discovers them, gasps at their appearance, and then breaks into laughter. Suddenly, Eloise and Josephine are belting out "Happy Birthday" to one of the stuffed animals on the ground, a giraffe. The unbridled happiness of four-year-olds gives me a jolt of ease that, with the help of my caffeine, has me in a better mood. Plus, I've finally got a good case today.

A baby has arrived in the NICU with something called a tracheo-esophageal fistula, which is an abnormal connection between the airway and the esophagus. Fixing this anomaly is one of my all-time favorite procedures in pediatric surgery, and the OR has given us clearance to go ahead and do it today. The operation is an elegant one that requires delicate hands and an intimate understanding of the complex physiology in these newborns. If the anesthesia or technical operation is executed poorly, the baby can easily decompensate on the table, meaning their oxygen levels plummet. If done perfectly, the baby will recover and be eating normally in less than a week.

I don my scrub cap and glasses and down a muffin before the case. Time to perform.

Scrubbing in at the sink before a case is one of my cherished surgical rituals. Some surgeons like to dry scrub with pure alcohol hand sanitizer, but I always do a wet scrub. Those few minutes are the moment when I set my intention for the procedure and slip into my zone. I rhythmically scrub my forearms and hands with the rough plastic bristles and feel the familiar lather. In the winter, sometimes my hands get so dry from all the scrubbing that I develop small, painful cracks in my skin. People who work in the OR learn all the best hand creams on the market. A bright green tub of O'Keeffe's Working Hands cream lives on my nightstand at home. I walk into the OR, hands dripping, and Cindy, our scrub, tosses me a towel. Cindy is a seasoned veteran in the OR. She knows how to keep all of the attendings calm and always has the right instruments prepared. It's going to be a good case.

We prep the baby, call a time-out for safety checks, and begin the operation. I carefully incise the baby's chest as my boss, the attending surgeon, and I swiftly identify the anatomical markers to dividing the fistula. There's the azygos vein, and right under that is the fistula. We encircle the offending connection to the airway and divide.

"Taking the fistula now," I say to the anesthesiologist.

Next, we find the upper pouch of the esophagus and bring it down just far enough to reach the other blind end. Finally, I sew the anastomosis, two corner stitches, three in the back row, knots on the inside, three on the front row, knots on the outside. I have the steps memorized by now. We leave a drain, close the chest, and get out. We're done in record time for me, under three hours.

"Look at that, Dr. Griggs. You're ready for the big leagues," my attending says, and smiles. Maybe he means it or maybe he just knows I need this lift right now. Either way, I'll take it.

I finish up the baby's procedure and see a string of text messages on my phone. No time to bask in the glory: there are three consults to see in the ED.

When I get to the emergency department, it's eerily quiet for midday, but the silence is pierced by a teenage girl, Maria, moaning on her stretcher, clutching her abdomen. A CT scan ordered by the ED earlier that morning shows horrible, perforated appendicitis. There is evidence of pus all over her abdomen and she's spiking a high fever with labs that show she's probably been battling this infection for a while already. Her Covid swab isn't back yet, so I don full protective gear. "Hi, I'm Dr. Griggs. I'm from the surgery team and I'm here to figure out how to help you, okay?" I explain. Teenagers are a tough population to treat, especially in New York City. These kids already have more street smarts than most adults will ever have. But inside, developmentally, they are still very much kids. Winning their trust is the key to helping them heal.

Maria tells me that she's been having belly pain on and off for two weeks and struggling to get by with Tylenol and Gatorade, but last night the pain got so bad that she couldn't take it anymore.

"You have a bad infection in your appendix," I explain. "Based on the CT scan I would say it's been ruptured for quite some time now. We need to bring you into the hospital for fluids, rest, and antibiotics."

Maria looks terrified.

"Do you want me to call your parents?" I ask.

"My parents don't live here," she answers. "I live with my aunt."

"Well, do you want me to call your aunt, then?"

Maria looks down. "You can't. She's . . . she's sick in the hospital too. She's got corona."

"I see," I respond. "I'm so sorry about that. But we're going to take good care of you here, all right? We're going to get you better. And we can try to get some updates on your aunt too. Can you give me her name?" I leave the room and rejoin my team and ask to get the social workers involved, which requires some logistical gymnastics given the number of people working remotely.

As we head upstairs, the ED resident runs to catch us. "Hey, just wanted to let you know that patient is Covid positive."

Ugh. Of course she is. "Thanks for letting me know."

At least we can start her on antibiotics now that she's here in the hospital. Finding her a bed upstairs, on the other hand, is going to be a challenge. Covid has disrupted our usual workflow and means the typical expected course of any disease process, even appendicitis, can be anything but predictable. I'm an expert by now at treating complicated appendicitis. In an otherwise healthy teenager, there's a protocol we usually follow by the book. But now, with her having Covid, I'm questioning everything I know, down to how much fluid to give this girl. We're all learning how to beat this monster on the fly.

When I get back to my office, someone knocks on the door and delivers me a new face shield. "Someone who works here has a family member who owns a 3D printing business and they figured out how to make these. Here you go, Doc."

I try it on. It's a little blurry and flimsy, but the gesture is so appreciated. Another little act of human kindness that goes a long way.

THURSDAY, APRIL 2

Eloise's nursery school in lower Manhattan is starting remote learning today. She's been so lucky to have my mom and Marsha, a professional in childhood learning, these last three weeks. But she doesn't understand why she isn't still with her fellow Sharks in the Blue Room of her school: a cozy den full of art supplies, books, a child-size kitchen, and fifteen other four- and five-year-olds. Eloise has just learned to write her name. Will she be able to continue to make progress by learning on a screen? How will my mom and Marsha and Pam do with supervising her remote learning? I feel guilty for not being there. When my mom isn't teaching her own students and helping with Eloise, she's potty training Jonah. At sixty-six, she didn't bank on having a second time around for these milestones. But I know I need her, Marsha's, and Pam's help, and that they're willing to give it.

I decide to email Eloise's teachers:

Hi Blue Room Teachers!

I was so excited to see and hear that distance learning has started today! I know it means so much to Eloise to see her teachers and her friends from school. Thank you for all the wonderful ideas and material you are putting together to entertain, teach, and give the children a stable sense of normalcy in these uncertain times!

I have what I hope is a small request. Would it be possible to include Marsha, Jill, and Pam on communications (especially those with action items!) from the classroom?

StoryPark is an amazing platform but for me right now, it's just a little cumbersome and difficult to keep up with everything. I get multiple StoryPark emails a day and I'm having trouble sorting through what the important, actionable items are (e.g. please order a calendar, weather cards, etc) and what is bonus programming (also awesome!). If it's not too much trouble, would it be possible to email me and Jill/Pam directly if there is something I should have sent to the house or organized for class? I want to stay in the loop but also have major overload of COVID-related emails from the hospital, in addition to operating and our normal clinical work and now helping on the adult side as well. I know this would require extra work for you guys and I don't want to overload anyone else either—but our family situation is a bit unique right now.

Additionally, I know most of the kids are getting lots and lots of time with their parents that they maybe don't normally get—but I hope you'll try to be sensitive to the fact that Eloise is away from both her Daddy AND her Mommy right now with no end in sight.

We quite literally don't know when it will be safe to visit because it would mean bringing all of our hospital exposures along with us. Eloise was doing great until the past couple of days when she has started asking me when she will be able to come back to NYC and if I will come pick her up ☹ This rips my heart out as you can imagine in what are already trying times at the hospital. I want to say that I know EVERYONE is going through tough times right now and I don't want it to seem like I am asking for special treatment. But I've learned it's important to ask for help when you need it—so I hope you'll consider the request.

Thank you so much again and hope everyone is staying safe.

Cornelia

Diane, her main teacher, writes back:

Dear Cornelia,

Thank you for reaching out! We most certainly want to help in any way! I am happy that Eloise is surrounded by supportive, loving people who will help her navigate this crazy, uncertain time—a time that has also taken her parents to the front lines . . . Eloise is resilient and understands when she needs extra love, attention, and support, and she will seek it out. That doesn't mean there won't be times when she is deeply sad and missing the two of you immensely, and that's okay. Eloise has such empathy for others and she knows that you aren't home because you are taking care of and helping people who are in need. She did the same thing, albeit on a much smaller and safer scale, with the sick babies in our classroom hospital. Eloise was always the doctor or parent diagnosing, treating, and soothing the patients. Eloise is full of love, understanding, and has a strong desire to help. However, knowing all that still makes it tough not to be with her more.

We will make sure to include everyone in our emails—I have added Jill and Marsha. As for StoryPark, you should be able to add any family member or caregiver to your account. You should also be able to change settings so that you are not getting notification emails from StoryPark. I know this will take a bit of time for you to do—maybe you can let your mom go into your StoryPark account (using your email and password) to change the settings for you. Unfortunately, I can't do it on my end.

Please, please reach out to us any time. As a team, we will be meeting to discuss thoughts on how we can better support Eloise and everyone around her during this time.

Thank you for your Eloise and for everything you are doing!

I realize, reading Diane's email, that teachers having to figure out new remote teaching methods, like StoryPark, is probably as stressful for them as it is for us at the hospital to have to figure out our new treatment protocols. Diane, like so many teachers, is fully devoted to her students and likely worried sick about figuring out how to take care of them and making sure that they don't fall behind. How can she know if her preschool class is still learning without being able to see the kids in person? Covid's toll on teachers is more invisible right now, but also heavy. *Typical*, I think, *that Covid is stealing the confidence and sapping the zeal of workers in the most women-led professions, nursing and teaching.*

FRIDAY, APRIL 3

My brother William texts me this morning to say he's been furloughed from his job. Just before the virus struck, we were celebrating his new position as the manager of a coffee and pastry chain in the city. The unemployment rate is skyrocketing to levels not seen since the Great Depression. William hasn't been able to reach anyone at the overburdened New York City unemployment office to file for benefits.

Anyone who comes to New York has to quarantine for fourteen days. "Social distancing" has become the phrase of the moment, and each day brings news of more cancellations: the baseball season, the summer Olympics, and almost every other large public event. Will's annual business trip to Austin, Texas, for SXSW is canceled. And we are the lucky ones.

Incredibly, the New York hospitals are still running out of PPE, and testing is nowhere near the scale it needs to be. At my hospital, hand sanitizer is now under lock and key and we've begun using improvised versions of it donated from distilleries. The latest version smells sickeningly similar to orange Creamsicles. While I am grateful to douse my hands in it, when the bootleg hand sanitizer dries, it feels like you've spilled sticky orange soda on your palms. I prefer full soap-and-water handwashing whenever possible.

I stay late at the hospital making rounds and at the end of the day I call Samantha, who is at home, to prep for the next day and talk about our list of patients, which is increasingly becoming one homogeneous list of children with Covid and related complications.

"I am starting to go nuts in my apartment," Samantha confesses. "I am truly scared to leave my house. I feel so alone. I've never felt this way, not even when I lived through war back at home. At least then I felt the comfort of my family."

Samantha grew up in eastern Congo and rarely lets down her guard like this: she is the polished and reserved one, while I am usually the hot-mess mom trying to juggle too much at once. Sam has become like a little sister to me at work this year, and my instinct is to look out for her. I've been so wrapped up in myself and my own fear that I've forgotten how much she must be suffering too.

"I wish I had more comforting words, Sam. New York has never felt so scary. The isolation at home is in some ways the worst part of it. I know coming to work has its own risks, but at least here you can be with people and feel useful. I know that's a weird silver lining, walking into the hospital—the place everyone else is trying to avoid at all costs. But you will feel better back at work in the morning, I'm almost certain."

Most things are better in the morning.

SATURDAY, APRIL 4

This morning I visit Jane in her office. She is defeated after a brutal overnight shift managing one of the pop-up Covid ICUs.

"They are all so scarily similar," Jane tells me of her patients. "And they are all going into renal failure. We seem to have just enough ventilators, but now we are running out of things like pumps for the feeding tubes and simple drugs for sedation. Their labs are the same. And they are So. Fucking. Sick, Cornelia. You look at them the wrong way and they code. Every time I come back from another shift, more of my patients are dead. Even the ones that you think are getting better . . . You get hopeful, you know? And then a few hours later they shit the bed. You want to give the families hope, but it's too sad. They are dying alone and it kills me. And there are a lot of people managing ventilators who just shouldn't be. I feel grateful that I did so much ICU training in fellowship because other people are completely out of their league. And many of the nurses are totally overwhelmed and scared."

I don't know what to say back. "I feel useless over here some-times," I confess. "I wish they would put me over on the adult side in the ICUs."

"No you don't." Jane scowls. "Trust me."

A part of me knows she's being protective. Another part of me feels like a coward. I have been reading up on the latest ICU proto-cols just in case. Experimental treatments like hydroxychloroquine and antivirals are being thrown at patients out of desperation. A drug called remdesivir is also being trialed in some of the sicker patients. But there's very little data to support any of this kitchen sink, throw-anything-and-everything-at-them approach. Despite all my studying, I know nothing could have prepared me for what Jane is going through. She is the true front line—or maybe the last line, depending on how you think about it.

Jane describes to me how one of the nurses combed her patient's hair before FaceTiming his family. A middle-aged Black man from the Bronx, he was overweight with prediabetes. Like so many patients, unsure of what to do, he had waited too long to come to the hospital. And by the time he got to the emergency room, he was gasping for air. He was quickly intubated and was now deteriorating on the ventilator. His chances of making it out alive were slim and the whole team knew it. He owned a bagel deli in Washington Heights and had a large family, and they had yet to come to terms with the inevitable. His nurse wanted him to look his best for the video call. It would probably be the last image his family saw of him.

"Most of the patient stories are similar," Jane explains with a note of exhaustion and despair. "They are mostly Latinx or Black, it seems. And, Cornelia, nothing we are doing over there seems to be working. Even the best and brightest ICU people seem hopeless. We're following ARDSNet protocols"—used in the ICU to treat respiratory failure—"but these Covid lungs, they can't take a joke. People are popping pneumos left and right. It's a total fucking cluster."

Jane and I both swear when we're frustrated. And I can tell she's gone to a dark place after this shift. "You really should go home and try to get some sleep," I suggest.

"Yeah, fucking right." Jane laughs. "When I try to sleep, all I hear are the vent alarms ringing in my ears. We're talking about silencing them because people are starting to lose their minds."

"Wow, that's dark," I respond. Turning off vent alarms would help protect the ICU teams' sanity, perhaps, but is a deeply gloomy sign of the ineffectiveness of our treatments. "Just get out of here today before you lose yours, okay?" I tell her. "I need you healthy to get through this thing." I mean that more than she knows. Jane is my lifeline without Rob and my kids here. Our friendship and solidarity are what keep me going.

"After I finish my notes," Jane replies.

SUNDAY, APRIL 5

Tonight is the first night I make it out of the hospital by 6:00 p.m. As I'm leaving I see a fifty-year-old woman on the sidewalk shrieking in Spanish into her cell phone outside the emergency room. I speak only a little bit of the language but can understand it well.

"He's gone! He's gone! The virus took my husband and now my baby too!" She's choking back her sobs. She is alone. I want to offer her something, a kind word, a tissue at least, but she hurries in the other direction. I collapse into tears on the way home in an Uber. The subways are running only limited hours and many people, myself included, are too scared to take it anyhow. My flimsy mask gets soaked with snot. The driver tells me it's okay—that all the nurses he brings home cry in the car at the end of their shifts.

When I make it home, as I change out of my dirty scrubs in my foyer, I hear it for the first time: the clapping. People are banging on pots and pans outside the window as the sun sets over the Hudson

River. I'm confused for a moment and then I realize that this is the clapping and pot banging I heard about from my friends and in the news. They are clapping for healthcare workers. They are clapping for us. I silently whisper a thank-you and go to take my much-needed hot shower.

My decontamination ritual is to strip down to my underwear when I get home. Then I carefully clean my phone and pager with bleach along with anything that has touched a hospital surface throughout the day. I leave my bag in the foyer—the "dirty" zone. Then I streak to the back of my apartment carrying my scrubs and the cloth cap I now wear over my hair all day. I throw everything in the laundry on the sanitary cycle. Then I shower. I let the water run burning hot and scrub everywhere with a foamy pink soap called Hibiclens. My favorite part is scraping underneath my short nails. Washing the day away has become my new therapy. For dinner I prepare a simple lentil soup from a can. I FaceTime the kids from home tonight instead of from the hospital, but they are busy with some craft project. I desperately miss the feeling of my toddlers rushing into my arms upon arriving home. I head to bed and try to avoid any more news about Covid for today. I can't handle it. Scrolling TikTok will do just fine.

I am still wrestling with the question *Is this what I signed up for?* In some ways, yes: I was always driven by a sense of altruism and self-sacrifice that accompanies a career in healthcare. Working every day to heal others, even when I feel tired and broken myself, is the essential component—the dogma, really, of our training. We tough it out. We know it's certainly worse to be in the patients' shoes. We hold each other up because only those who work in healthcare can truly understand the special kind of sacrifice our work involves. Of course, many other fields require sacrifice and some more than healthcare. But my friend Marian, a seasoned ICU nurse, explains it best: "Covid feels like being a firefighter running into a burning house with no gear or equipment." For other professionals whose daily work requires heroic acts of bravery, such as firefighters and members of the military, that instinctual reflex to save a life at your own risk is often accompanied by years of training and many layers of protective gear and armor. We don't have the training for a global pandemic, which isn't such a surprise, but it's the lack of meaningful protective gear that is the real kicker. I sound like a broken record when I tell my friends. It feels like only the healthcare workers here on the ground can really appreciate the outrage we feel.

But here it is, flaring up again. We didn't sign up to live apart from our children and spouses for weeks on end with no clear guidance on proper home decontamination protocols for transitioning to reuniting. My friend Dan, an anesthesiologist, told me he was living in a trailer in his driveway. Another friend of mine in thoracic surgery sees his son only by waving through a window on his backyard porch. Jane is living in her damp basement.

I try to remember what grounds me: the sense of duty I feel to my patients and colleagues. Among the most inspiring to me is Valeria, who shows up every day to work in the environmental services department. She continues to clean our offices daily and restocks all of the supplies we need to keep the surfaces around us Covid-free. Valeria and other environmental services workers are underappreciated and too often unseen. She makes roughly $15 an hour. She seems relatively unfazed by the current chaos, but maybe it's a brave act. Still, her soothing and determined presence never cracks. I know she's supporting her family here in New York and routinely sends money back to her family members in the Dominican Republic as well. Valeria's son is in college at an Ivy League school and she loves to brag about him and show me pictures. She hopes he will go into medicine. If there is a part of her that wants to run far away from this place, as I do, she never lets it show. This kind of sacrifice and dedication from the other healthcare workers around me is what fuels me. I may not have signed up for this, but that doesn't mean I am going to give up and stay home.

MONDAY, APRIL 6

"Mommy, will you come pick me up?" Eloise pleads over FaceTime. It guts me. I want nothing more than to rush to Connecticut and pull my children into my arms, to bury my face in the comforting smell of their little toddler heads.

"Oh, lovey, I so wish I could. But Mommy still has to clean up some more germs at the hospital," I tell her, trying to smile but choking back the urge to cry.

Eloise nods and doesn't fight me, doesn't throw a tantrum, just runs off to play and hands the phone back to my mom. "Just remember it's so much harder for you than it is for them," my mom gently comforts me.

I hope my kids won't remember much from this time. So far they really do seem mostly happy and unaffected by the pandemic. They spend their days making up games and puppet shows and are surrounded by loving, attentive adults. They have so much more than most other children do. But it still kills me to hear Eloise begging to be picked up so she can come home. While other children have seen more of their parents in the past few weeks than possibly at any other time in their lives, my children have been temporarily but functionally orphaned by Covid. Today I am feeling really sorry for my little family.

In Boston, Rob has been operating on emergency surgery patients nonstop, both for those who have Covid and those who don't. Even though his elective practice is shut down, he is still one of the few surgeons manning the slots for true surgical disasters that cannot wait. Luckily, the supply of PPE is more plentiful in Boston, and Rob's N95 gets cleaned and decontaminated every night. But the hospitals in Boston, like New York, are still overflowing with Covid ICU patients.

The lucky ones avoid ventilators, skirting by with just some supplemental oxygen. Many get intubated, rapidly decompensate, and die swiftly. Others linger and suffer and slowly get sicker and sicker. At this point it seems like we're in for a long ride and we are all just learning to cope. The death rate from Covid in New York is still high—about six hundred each day—and we're not sure it has peaked yet.

I can't fall asleep at night. The ambulance sirens are haunting and quite literally continuous. Sometimes I can hear two at once. Body after body is being rushed to the hospital.

Downtown Manhattan is like a ghost town. There are signs on

almost every store: OUR STORE IS TEMPORARILY CLOSED. LET'S FIGHT THE SPREAD OF COVID-19 TOGETHER. Grocery stores, pharmacies, and of course the wine and liquor stores are open.

In the hospital, we have run out of dialysis and feeding tube machines. That means the time I feared of us having to ration care is actually here. Doctors and nurses have to pick and choose who has the best shot at surviving and deny the necessary equipment to other patients. No one wants to talk about it, but it is happening.

CNN and other news outlets even catch wind of a departmental message from one of our renowned and revered pediatric cardiac surgeons. Dr. B. is a God in the world of heart surgery. They have published parts of his letter: "We have had to ration care and make decisions about who is considered an urgent or emergent case. . . . The lack of Personal Protective Equipment is infuriating, such a symbolic failure. Already, the system is so overwhelmed that we have run out of our most basic protective gear. Who would have thought that a simple plain surgical mask, something we use and discard multiple times a day during normal times, would become a rationed product in world-famous hospitals??"

With Dr. B.'s team down to a single operating room, they have had to delay countless urgent procedures for babies with serious cardiac illnesses—shunt-dependent infants, children with ventricular septal defects in heart failure, teenagers with bad valves. Their families are stuck in an infuriating waiting game, wondering how sick their child will have to be to warrant one of the rare emergency operating slots.

The limited availability of dialysis machines means that some patients with severe Covid are being pushed to the furthest limits of kidney failure. Dr. O. is now one of those patients. He's become so sick that he is now one of the few adult patients on ECMO. Jane was on call the night his condition started to rapidly deteriorate. She could barely speak the morning after. Thankfully, there was an ECMO machine available. The entire department is even more on pins and needles lately, knowing how close one of our own—a true legend in our field—is to death.

The ban on visitors is one of the hardest changes to cope with. Patients are dying in isolation from their families, which feels extraordinarily cruel. There are closets crammed full of their belongings because no family members are allowed to come pick them up. Before Covid, we made every effort to let patients die with dignity, with loved ones at their side and religious services of their choice. In the ICU we would go to great lengths to rid people of tubes and wires so that wives could kiss their husbands goodbye. We'd arrange platters of food and quiet rooms to grieve. All of that is gone now.

The lack of visitors puts even more pressure and guilt on the staff to provide humane care despite the barriers of our masks and gowns. But it's impossible. Instead of doubling down on human connection, many of us withdraw into ourselves. "For the first time in my career," Jane admits to me sorrowfully, "I am having trouble remembering my patients' names."

For elderly patients with Covid who are so frail that there is practically no chance for survival, sometimes the most compassionate thing we can do is transition them to comfort measures and help them die as quickly and peacefully as possible instead of prolonging their suffering. There is a sense of urgency to help their families come to terms with the inevitable and support this process. It's a hard truth, but it frees up a ventilator or a room for a patient who actually has a prayer of making it through.

Rob is beginning to witness firsthand another, stealthier side of the health dangers Covid poses. The delay Covid is causing to more routine care for patients will have devastating consequences for years to come. It will be nearly impossible to measure the lives lost due to a missed colonoscopy or mammogram, the undiagnosed minor stroke or heart attack. Rob's practice was once busy with cancer patients needing semi-urgent surgery, but now he's only doing emergency surgeries. The backlog of cancer patients who are having to hold off on nonemergency treatment is a huge concern.

I worry about what Rob's own past chemotherapy means for his immune system. He doesn't. He's happy to be seen, especially by those who don't know what he's been through, as a fit guy in his mid-thirties, straight out of training and eager to help. Rob somehow has been spared from the crippling anxiety I am feeling many days. Maybe it's because he has stared down death before; maybe it's because I'm an overthinker. But showing up every day just seems easier for him. "I'm going to be fine, babe," he reassures me daily.

At least Boston has had almost two weeks of lead time to be

better prepared, and the city is littered with excellent hospitals. New York City, on the other hand, has seen a huge decline in the number of available hospital beds over the past decade, along with a surge in retail clinics and for-profit urgent care centers.

The 2010 closing of St. Vincent's Hospital in downtown Manhattan is emblematic of this shift. Perched in the heart of the West Village, St. Vincent's was the receiving hospital for the survivors of the *Titanic* in 1912, at the forefront of treating patients during the AIDS epidemic in the eighties, and the triage site for many of those injured in the World Trade Center attacks in 2001. But the rich history of the hospital was not enough to save it from financial ruin stemming from management problems and the shifting economics of operating in a building in downtown Manhattan. There is now an urgent care center that sits near the site of the former hospital, and it has no ability to handle the kind of acuity we are seeing during Covid. The situation is even worse in other neighborhoods in the outer boroughs, where struggling hospitals that once served the undocumented and uninsured, like Interfaith Medical Center in Bedford-Stuyvesant, have been shut down over the previous decades. Medical deserts are what we have there now.

When I first started seriously thinking about becoming a doctor, my biggest dream was to open a free clinic at a place called the Northern Dispensary, a funny triangular-shaped building near the former St. Vincent's. I would often stroll by it, peering into the cloudy windows, through which I could see the shapes of the old dental equipment that was still left over from the late 1980s when the building was last used. The local lore was that there was a stipulation on the deed of the building that required it to be used for the medical care of New York's "worthy poor."

At one point I even had a friend who worked in real estate do some digging around and research for me, just out of curiosity. Apparently it was owned by a real estate magnate who owned historic downtown properties and I believe was just sitting on them. When Rob and I first started dating, whenever we passed the Northern Dispensary, I would point to it in youthful ambition. "I'm going to buy it one day and turn it into a free clinic for kids!" I told him.

Less than a year later, Rob proposed to me outside the steps of the building. "Your dreams are now my dreams too," he promised.

But as I would learn, a free clinic was a pipe dream unless I found a wealthy, benevolent sponsor to fund it. And in the years that followed our engagement, just getting through training and keeping our little family intact proved so challenging that big dreams like the Northern Dispensary were put on the back burner. *Maybe one day,* I would still occasionally think before Covid.

Now those kinds of dreams are far from my mind. All I can think about is making it out of this hellscape intact.

SATURDAY, APRIL 11

Thinking of my commitment to speak out and report on what I'm seeing, I've posted a tweet about a medical trainee in the city who may have died from Covid. I know that there is another on ECMO. Outside of New York, confirmed reports of nurses, doctors, paramedics, medical trainees, and other first responders dying from Covid are cropping up all over the country. I've seen the memorial pages in their honor.

In my tweet, I suggested that some attending physicians are benefiting from the current arrangement where residents and fellows are stuck cross-covering the EDs and ICUs while high-salaried specialists are cloistered in their homes. "Medical trainees like me signed up to save lives, not to be a shield," I wrote. Residents and fellows are not only paid lower salaries and work eighty hours a week or more but have more Covid exposure and risk than their supervisors and bosses, who are paid four or five times as much while working fewer hours. The attendings cover one or maybe two shifts a week while the residents work twelve-hour shifts with only four days off a month. In non-Covid times, this is just part of the process of medical training. But to me the risk that Covid poses to the lives of every healthcare worker changes the deal.

One of my residents, Maddie, has a six-month-old at home and her nanny just quit. Her husband is struggling to do his tech job from home with a crying infant on his lap, and her marriage and sanity are both on the brink of collapse. I sent Maddie home for the week to try to sort out her childcare situation. My other resident, Jake, has grown a mangy beard and looks as if he's lost twenty pounds. Everywhere around me I see residents buckling under the weight and the pressure of the pandemic.

———

A surgeon from the adult side of the hospital is now coming after me. He fires back to my tweet that I have been "MIA" as far as he can tell.

I don't know where he got the idea that I'm MIA. Maybe because I haven't been redeployed to the adult ICU. But I am already working the max number of hours allowed every week, usually more, and treating middle-aged adults on the children's side.

My bitterness over the inequality and unfairness that I perceive happening between supervisors and residents wasn't meant to include attendings like Jane, who are busting their butts in the ICU. But she, too, took offense and told me as much. I feel bad about that, and it makes me wonder if I was wrong. But even Jane has much more ability to leverage her status and benefits to protect herself and her family than a trainee. I know this because Rob is a first-year attending like Jane and I've seen his contract. Rob and Jane have life and disability insurance and protections in place for their families if they die or develop significant, long-term injuries on the job.

My tweet was about doctors in training, but the nurses, of course, are experiencing an even worse imbalance of power and responsibility. Especially in the ICU, they have to physically enter Covid-positive rooms much more frequently than physicians do. My friend Krista, an ICU nurse, tells me, "Every shift I am at least doubled, if not more. And the docs are just hiding behind their computers." Doubled means that she is taking care of two to three times as many patients at once as compared to pre-Covid times. Usually the ICU has a 1:1 nursing-to-patient ratio. "Some of the residents refuse to go in the rooms," she says. "And they have no idea how to manage a vent or titrate a drip. It makes me want to scream." Krista was already on the verge of quitting before the pandemic. She's a talented nurse but she has no tolerance for what she perceives as abuse.

———

All of this adds up to the feeling that the moment when we were all united as healthcare workers against a common cause has come and gone. Our hospital administrators' daily updates have taken on a strict and unsympathetic tone, perhaps in reaction to the influx of angry emails they are receiving from staff. In a live video update, a top-level administrator said: "Please, for you and your families, stop sending emails, cards, and letters saying that we are disrespecting you. If you feel that way, we can understand that. You're entitled to your opinion. It raises for us whether you, in fact, want to keep working [here]. I'm not gonna continue to harp on that, but I ask you, really, you have to make your own judgments."

The video went public. Now a Change.org petition is circulating for this administrator's removal because she is perceived as threatening hospital staff with professional retaliation for expressing that they feel disrespected. Tensions could not be higher.

———

Some of the residents at another hospital in the city are calling for hazard pay, which seems totally appropriate given the dire circumstances. A letter from one of their senior urologists is now circulating on Twitter: "I have been involved in the interview process for our medical school. . . . I would like each and every one of you to reflect on your answer to the following scenario: Your medical community is engaged in an all hands on deck effort to provide care during a pandemic. In the midst of this effort, would you sign a petition for hazard pay? Your response to this interview scenario should guide your actions today." His chastising words are causing a flurry of outrage among the medical Twitterverse. "This is so wrong on every level and is textbook abuse of power and gaslighting, amongst other malignancies," one surgeon writes. I agree with her.

But I also feel guilty. At times I wonder if my millennial generation really is weaker than my parents' and grandparents' generations, which protested and fought for major civil rights changes and built a huge economy following World War II. This is not the first time millennial doctors have been called out for complaining, and I've personally been called a "privileged snowflake" before. But I think what it comes down to is that my peers and I tend to have a different value system. We prize overall well-being, the quality of our lives outside the hospital, and home-life integration. Surgical training programs used to joke and brag about the high divorce rates among their trainees. The culture is changing now, albeit slowly, by adopting a more modern approach to well-being in and outside of the workplace. Increasingly, people recognize that the increased rates of addiction, depression, anxiety, burnout, and suicide are unsustainable in our profession.

I remind myself that everyone I know does think I am tough. I operated through two pregnancies and took minimal maternity leave. I was back on call just three weeks after Eloise was born. I took my general surgery board exam during the worst of Jonah's infant colic at six weeks old. I know I can do hard things.

Sometimes I am able to convince myself that I am lucky to be here. Truthfully, I am honored to play even a small role in the story of fighting this pandemic, and I know that I'm living through a part of history that I'll remember forever. I also feel lucky to have a job. But when my peers and friends in other professions are given months longer maternity leaves, routine bonuses, and other major work perks, sometimes I'm left to wonder if those of us in medicine have given up too much for too long.

Is a little hazard pay really too much to ask for?

———

I decide to block the surgeon who has come after me on Twitter. One of my dear friends from Boston is now texting me that this guy is well-known as a "royal jerk." Apparently, he regularly posts and brags about his extravagant cigar collection. "It's coming up on 5pm—which one should I hit tonight?" says a post from the surgeon that my friend sends to me as a screenshot. "Coming after a resident on Twitter is a bad look and he should know better," my friend writes.

"Thanks, friend," I write back.

Thankfully, the public relations team at the hospital is in my corner. They see value in my tweets and in having someone from the medical staff—a young woman, no less—present a public face to the community. While some senior attendings are annoyed by my public comments and media appearances, I've decided I will continue to speak out. But I also realize that I have to accept that there can be long-term consequences if I want to keep posting my thoughts on social media. I decide that I need to control my anger and do my best not to sound self-righteous.

After working for Mehmet Oz, I have my eyes open to the downsides of seeking fame. But celebrity is truly not what I'm looking for here. There are still plenty of Americans who want to believe doctors like me are using scare tactics and creating a mythical boogeyman out of Covid for our own profit and gain. We have created a healthcare system so complex and so unwieldy that most people don't have or even know a doctor that they trust anymore. I don't even have a primary care doctor for myself. I haven't had my lipids checked in over a decade, and I'm a surgeon! Our healthcare system has pivoted away from providing personalized, high-quality primary and preventive care. In doing so, we have sacrificed and eroded a lot of public trust in the name of profit. People struggle to be seen for their most basic health needs. Mothers across the country are getting price gouged with enormous hospital bills just for giving birth. Our government has made following basic common sense and human decency into a political mud-wrestling match. It's no wonder that the public doesn't know who to believe anymore. If people can find something emotional or relatable in me and the stories I publicize, maybe I can help get the messaging right.

Before letting go of my anger entirely, I decide to call one of my friends who works closely with the surgeon baiting me on Twitter. I'm paranoid that the entire surgery department now thinks I'm just an attention whore. Maybe she can give me some perspective.

"Listen, not every tweet is going to land," she tells me.

Sometimes it is that simple.

SUNDAY, APRIL 12

There are more of the white refrigerator morgue trucks parked to the side of the main entrance of the hospital. I see them as I take my morning walk to Starbucks. I keep picturing the piles of corpses.

In learning to cope with the present circumstances, I have gone mostly numb to how awful this all is. Covid Land is my new normal. It feels like I am functioning on autopilot every day, operating and rounding and taking care of sick children as if this is all normal, and the only difference is the mask.

Talking to my colleagues helps bring me back to the reality of what is going on. My friend Anna is a widely respected ICU nurse on the adult side. She used to help me when I was a junior resident in the ICU during my first two years of residency, when I was still learning the ropes. She has been taking care of Covid patients since they first started arriving and is one of the nurses assigned to Dr. O., who remains critically ill. Being surrounded by the best of the best at the hospital hasn't been enough. If we lose him, it will be a huge blow to morale. He is truly irreplaceable. I shiver to think of all the children and adults who won't be saved by his miraculous surgical skill.

When I ask Anna how she's doing, her response shows her incredible strength but also how much she's had to push aside in order to stay focused, especially during the most "chaotic" times of the first few days and weeks. She says, "I just felt like so much was happening at the same time. I don't know how I got my thoughts together. The turnover was so fast. It was so intense and so much. I don't panic. I don't go into disarray. But that first week I had to step outside and cry. I prayed and said, 'Oh my God, is this really happening?'"

Visibly distressed, Anna describes calling families to get their permission and consent to place tubes and catheters on her patients. "When you call to get consent from these families . . . the conversations are just 'I can't see him? How is he doing? Is he still okay?' And your conversation goes from consent to saying, 'He's very sick . . . You can call as much as you want and ask for me and I will update you as much as I can.' It's so sad because I have to cut those conversations short to take care of other things. It's such a disservice because they are not able to see or speak to these patients . . . to their family. And I felt like from their end they kinda knew this might be the last time they see their parents or loved one. I carry that with me."

It is unnerving to see even someone as unshakable as Anna clearly shaken. "I had the luxury that I lost my dad at home, with his family and my mom surrounded by loved ones," she explained. "I call that a luxury because . . . it's very hard to paint a picture for the families when you know they're not going to make it."

Somehow Anna is also managing to supervise two kids at home who are doing school online. Plus, her husband has recently recovered from Covid. Her two siblings are also nurses. "We're like soldiers called to battle." She laughs. But she says the moment things got real was the night in the third week of March when the ICU doubled its patient census overnight. "We went from ten patients to twenty over the span of twelve hours. And then by six or seven o'clock, four of those admissions died. In less than two hours. The fellow and I kept going from one room to another room. We were tag-teaming who was calling the family, helping write the death notes, pronouncing the patients. When I went home I cried and I cried and I prayed and I cried. Just praying fervently that somehow, whatever we're supposed to learn at this moment—'whatever's up there for us to learn or whatever you're trying to teach us'—I hope we could learn. I cried myself to sleep and then I had to work that same night again."

She does her rosary before every shift, she tells me. "I talked about end of life with my husband: 'You know what you have to do if and when this happens to me. Do not ECMO. Do not VAD [ventricular assist device]. DNR [do not resuscitate]. I do not want that if there is no life for me and if there is no purpose of my life.

You already know what to do.' He knows me to be stubborn. He's known this already before Covid."

Even Anna, who has worked the toughest and sickest units in this giant New York City hospital, has never witnessed death on this scale in her entire career. Truly, none of us have even imagined a tragedy of this scope.

"It's such a discrepancy, what you see in the news," Anna goes on. "These people are not elderly. We are losing people in their thirties. I just lost one last night."

I want to hug her, but those small gestures of comfort remain off-limits at the hospital. Instead I simply thank her for everything she's doing in one of the most brutal roles in the building.

I check in on my friend Alex later that day. His hospital still won't let him get back to work because he continues to test positive for Covid after more than a month. Emotionally, he is a wreck. Ally has moved out.

"I've never hated anyone so much before, Cornelia," Alex tells me.

"Maybe you will actually love being a parent?" I timidly suggest.

"I will do what I have to do. My happiness is irrelevant now," he says.

The pandemic has exposed cracks in the relationships of many couples I know. Several of my friends are now teetering on divorce. Apparently in China the divorce rate has also surged.

Alex wants to fly to New York to pitch in here but his job won't let him come. "Can't lose my job; then I'm even less help," he says.

His specialty in cardiac ECMO will be needed where he is soon enough, I fear, if Covid begins to surge in his part of the country as predicted. With the baby due in just a couple of months, I hope I am wrong. I hope that Alex and my medical friends across the country are spared the disaster scenario that is happening here.

THURSDAY, APRIL 16

My friend Jamie, a nurse in the ED, has admitted four of her colleagues today. "This is different," she tells me. "These are my friends and the people I work with every day."

After trying to tough out their coughs and fevers at home, all of them came stumbling into the ED, looking for help when their breathing worsened. For Jamie, seeing her colleagues on the other side of the curtain is deeply disturbing. "All I can do is keep checking in on them and hope," she says.

My medical school friend Hadi, who is now a cardiologist at a different hospital in New York City, writes a missive on Facebook: "Oxygen rounds is a new term I have become all too familiar with. I have a hospital full of medications . . . but the only truly effective medicine we have is oxygen. We blow it at high flow rates into people's mouths and nostrils, a crutch to help the lungs that are struggling and staggering. And it's in shorter supply than I would like. It flows forever from spigots on the wall, but we have many times more patients on stretchers that line hallways further and further from the spigots on the walls. We place portable tanks next to stretchers, but the tanks run out and we can't refill them fast enough. Once per hour, sometimes twice, I walk the halls, hunting for gauges approaching empty and hoping the cabinet holds a replacement. Invariably, I find empty ones and hope it hasn't been empty long. Invariably someone is turning blue. It's no one's fault. It's everyone's fault. It's Covid's fault. And there just aren't enough eyes and hands to keep up. I mutter a promise to check three times next hour."

Everywhere I look, I see another colleague in despair. And while healthcare workers are getting sick, overwhelmingly our patients are coming from the most vulnerable communities in the city. The despair that healthcare workers feel is just a small fraction of the despair among the families who are losing multiple relatives to Covid. Neighborhoods like the South Bronx and central Queens, areas of Brooklyn that are the so-called food and medical deserts wedged right next to some of the nation's wealthiest zip codes, are being brutally ravaged by this virus. Meanwhile there are protests against wearing masks and social-distancing restrictions in states like Michigan, Kentucky, and Oklahoma. I can only imagine that staying inside feels foolish for those who can't see and touch and witness how savage and cruel this virus can be. But the president's insistence on opening up the country is way too premature. We cannot afford to simply bulldoze our way through the pandemic for political gain. Too many have already died unnecessarily. If we simply lift all of the protections now, the human cost will be unbearable. In some ways it already is.

I'm particularly sensitive about the idea of lifting protections at this critical juncture because it finally feels like maybe, just maybe, we are starting to turn a corner, and it would be foolish to risk jeopardizing that. The total number of Covid patients in the hospital has been going down this week. The hospital is predicting that we are past the peak. The ICUs are still overflowing with patients on ventilators, but some patients are making it out alive. The USNS *Comfort* and the Javits Center, temporarily transformed into a make-shift hospital, finally started taking Covid-positive patients a week ago. I don't want to get ahead of myself, but it looks like there may be reason to be optimistic for some kind of relief after the surge. With my birthday approaching in a few days, it would be nice to feel a measure of hope.

FRIDAY, APRIL 17

Last week, I found out that Rob and I will both be off the weekend before my birthday, which is April 22. We debated back and forth about meeting up in Connecticut, neither of us knowing if we would pose a real infectious risk to my parents and the kids. Interstate travel is technically not even allowed by either of our hospitals.

But it's been five weeks since I've seen the kids, and eight since I've seen Rob. It's longer than I ever imagined I could possibly endure, but I'm losing my mind. Rob and I talk and decide to bite the bullet. We take measure of the risk and decide it's worth it to our family to make a visit to Connecticut. So many of our other doctor friends have started to loosen up their protocols at home and are now living among their families as they did before Covid while being extra careful about changing clothes, washing hands, and showering once they get home from the hospital. So far, no one we know of has infected their kids or family members by bringing Covid home from work.

Rob comes all the way down from Boston on Friday the seventeenth to pick me up and then we drive together to Connecticut. It's so good to see him, but on the way I somehow became fixated on a worry that the kids will not be excited to see us. Despite FaceTiming them every day, my anxious thoughts have me convinced that my children have lost their sense of attachment to us as parents.

Rob reassures me that it's not going to happen. We talk about how our world has changed so much in the weeks since my mom left with them. So many mundane things I took for granted now feel risky. Even going to get the groceries is a calculated exercise in risk mitigation. Kay recently sent me a funny meme mocking the stereotypical New York City mom, who used to avoid chemicals near her children at all costs and only shopped for whole, organic foods. "Now we clean their apples with a Lysol wipe," the punch line read.

It's not even that funny, especially when the president seems to have casually suggested exploring injection of household disinfectant as a treatment for Covid. Was he joking? Even if he was, the total and utter absurdity and chaos of this moment makes it impossible to ignore the recklessness of that kind of comment. Numerous doctors have spoken up to clarify that injecting bleach or Lysol is poisonous. There is genuine concern that Americans will attempt to do it. Just when you think this pandemic cannot get any more twisted, it takes a new and absurd turn.

As usual, Sarah Cooper won the day with her classic lip syncs. She's my favorite Twitter comedian right now. All she has to do is mouth the president's exact words and the absolute absurdity is so tragic that you can't do anything but laugh. This is real life. Her performances are helping us process how upside down everything feels.

I wonder how much of this Eloise and Jonah have processed. Kids are so emotionally intelligent, it would be impossible for them not to pick up and absorb the anxiety of the adults around them. I don't want them to grow up thinking the world is a bad and scary place. But in order to convince them that we are safe, I am going to have to believe it too.

We arrive at my parents' house and execute my crazy decontamination plan. Rob and I take turns rinsing off in the outdoor shower, which typically doesn't get used except in the summer. The chilly April New England air is not pleasant. We scrub with the Hibiclens that I've brought and change into fresh clothes before entering the house. We both agree that we will go in without masks. We are asymptomatic and have been as careful as we can be.

Eloise and Jonah are watching their favorite cartoon, *Octonauts*, when we walk in. And then: bliss. The kids miraculously break from their show and fling their bodies into our arms. Jonah's hair has grown into a shaggy mop. I could swear Eloise looks taller. We all pile onto the couch and collapse in a happy heap to enjoy an afternoon of Netflix cartoons. This is all I've wanted for weeks. When it's time

.to put Jonah down for his nap, Rob and I fight over who gets to do it. Normally, we'd bicker over who *has* to do it. Jonah has never been a good sleeper, and getting him to nap on the weekends is a battle that can sometimes turn into an hour-long exercise in toddler negotiations. Today I say: bring on the tantrum. This is the normal stuff of everyday life that I have missed so much.

Jonah and I go upstairs and read three books. He turns the pages of his favorite early-words board book and points to a pair of pants. "Jonah's pants." He giggles to himself wildly, clearly an inside joke that I've missed out on in the intervening weeks since we last read together. I sing Jonah his songs, rock him in the glider, and gently place him down in the portable crib. He burrows under the blankets and covers his face with three loveys. I lie down on the bed in the same room and drift off into a long nap myself, the first truly restful sleep I've had in weeks.

Thirty-seven sounds so much older than thirty-six. I'm now in my late thirties. When I started surgical residency as a twenty-eight-year-old, I remember calculating what my age would be when I graduated and was horrified at how terrifyingly old thirty-seven seemed. Now here I am, about to be a full-fledged pediatric surgeon, with two kids, a husband, a golden retriever, and a mortgage on a condo in Boston. I used to fear becoming boring and predictable. But after the last decade, it would be a welcome change of pace.

The younger me would probably think I am just giving up. I can still vividly channel the girl in her mid- to late twenties who was living her best life as a medical student in New York City. I had a gaggle of close friends, was the social chairman of my med school class, and somehow had the stamina to try every brand-new pop-up restaurant while pulling all-nighters before my exams and hospital shifts. Those were my glory days of underground karaoke bars in the East Village and concerts at Brooklyn Bowl, where my brother Will helped staff the talent.

When I started residency, things began to shift. Soon my wildest fantasy was a night of uninterrupted sleep. Friend meet-ups happened mostly at playgrounds with large coffees in hand. When I wasn't in my stereotypical uniform of scrubs and a Patagonia fleece with the hospital logo embroidered on the sleeve, fashion became an oversized sweater with leggings. Just before Covid, I would regularly scoff at the sceney brunch crowd lined up in front of Bubby's near our apartment. The food is decent, but who in their right mind waits outside in the cold for thirty-dollar eggs and Bloody Marys you can make just as well at home? I've arrived. I am officially that lame old grumpy lady. I don't deserve to be in New York. That's okay with me.

SATURDAY, APRIL 25

BEEP. BEEP. BEEP. My pager blares at 4:00 p.m. from the waist-band of my scrubs and I startle at the abrupt break in the silence of my office. I drop an oily forkful of lettuce from my sad cafeteria salad onto my scrub pants as I reach to unholster the pager. A reflexive combination of annoyance and curiosity washes over me as I read the words on the screen: "Baby Nia oxygen requirement now 100%, sats plummeting, can we discuss?" "Sats" means how much oxygen is in her blood.

Shit. Shit. Shit. Nia is a new Covid admit to the PICU, trans-ferred in from another hospital this morning because they were worried she would need ECMO. She is less than a month old, one of my youngest patients yet to have Covid, and has already been intubated with respiratory distress.

Here we go.

I reach for the phone to call my resident, Caleb, to get an update.

My skin is parched and flaking from scrubbing myself each night with surgical soap. I barely sleep anymore. I'm like a walking raw nerve: exposed, strung out, and twitchy. I have a mountain of notes to write and am just getting to my lunch in the late afternoon, and now putting a sick baby on ECMO means I'm going to be stuck here at the hospital after hours. Again.

Then the perpetual guilt kicks in: *How can I whine about working late when someone's child is crashing?*

"Saw your text. How bad is the gas?" I ask Caleb.

"It's really shitty. Her pH is now less than 7.2," he responds.

"I'm on my way up."

Nia's mother has struggled on and off with addiction and she had almost no prenatal care throughout her pregnancy. But as far as we know, Nia was born perfectly healthy and full-term. Nia and her mother have been living in a Covid shelter, a homeless shelter specifically dedicated to Covid-positive individuals. I'm embarrassed to admit that I didn't even realize such places existed. I can't help but think of my friends cozied up in their second homes upstate or in the Hamptons, complaining about hunkering down and not being able to socialize with friends. Even those of us in the hospital are lucky by comparison. I can't comprehend the depths of cruelty that people living in poverty during the pandemic are facing.

The elevator dings and I turn in to the NICU, scanning my badge at the door. The typically bustling lobby is a ghost town. It's so creepy here that I even miss Jerry, the curmudgeonly guard usually sitting at the desk who yells at me for trying to sneak my coffee into the nursery. "NO OUTSIDE FOOD OR DRINKS ALLOWED," he barks, clearly getting satisfaction in cutting the surgeons down a bit at every chance. Only the staff who are absolutely required to keep the patients alive are here now.

Caleb is standing outside Nia's room. Nurses—four of them, it looks like—are attending to the baby. I can hear from the pitch of the monitor by Nia's crib that her oxygen is dangerously low. Some of the sickest children are flipped around so that their heads are at the feet of their beds, and Nia is one of them. This allows for easier access to the area we need to reach to do ECMO in an emergency. I always know the names of the children in the hospital in this position.

Caleb explains: "They just did her cares and now they can't get her sats above 90. They're maxed out on nitric and her peak pressures are sky-high. There's a new ABG cooking." In other words, Nia is crashing and her system can't get enough oxygen despite maximum support from the ventilator. I pull up Nia's chart to assess her most recent chest X-ray. It looks horrible. There's barely any aerated lung; the whole thing is a cloudy mess. It's all gummed up. The NICU has started medication to support her blood pressure, an ominous sign.

"Call the perfusionists," I tell Caleb. "We're going to have to go on ECMO."

I call my boss to tell him he needs to drive in to supervise. He doesn't question me. "I'll be there in fifteen minutes," he responds.

I call Nia's mother. Her cell service is spotty and her whereabouts are somewhat unclear, but I'm required to ensure that her mother's consent for the procedure is "informed." I'm thankful that this isn't the NICU's first conversation with her about the risk and potential need for ECMO. I explain over the phone how dire the situation is, how we're going to do everything we can to save Nia's life. I carefully explain the risks and benefits of ECMO in matter-of-fact terms. And I promise we're going to take good care of her. On the other end of the line, she gives a detached "Okay."

"Just to clarify, does that mean I have your permission to put Nia on ECMO?" I ask.

"Yes, Doctor," she replies, her voice still sounding like it's floating in from another planet.

"Okay, I will update you as soon as we're done. If you're not able to make it here, I will call you on this line."

As soon as the paperwork is settled, I scrub in. Nia's head is at the foot of her tiny hospital bed. There's a large roll under her little shoulders to stretch out her neck vessels for easier dissection. In any children's hospital the providers would know this as the ECMO-ready position for a child under 30 kilograms or so.

Caleb preps Nia's chest and neck with Betadine, the orangey-brown liquid we use to cleanse all the bacteria off the skin before surgery. The rule in surgery is to prep widely, just in case you need to extend your incision or perform an emergency maneuver. When we go on ECMO, I always prep the chest in case we need swift access to the heart. I confirm that our whole team is ready and then the room pauses in near silence for a time-out. My attending signals me to go ahead and do the procedure on my own with Caleb. Once everything is ready, we begin. I have Caleb make a tiny incision just above Nia's clavicle. Her tissues are paper thin, and I spread out the filmy layer of neck muscles to expose the critical vessels of her neck. Next, I show Caleb how to swiftly encircle the carotid artery and jugular vein. Like two small strands of wet spaghetti, the vessels pulse and throb below our instruments. After getting control of the vessels, I ask Caleb to make a small puncture in the vein, which is particularly fragile. His hand quivers as he makes the nick, and I furtively move my hand to steady his. Next, it's time to place the first cannula.

"When I let up my traction, gently twist, and point the cannula just slightly towards the heart," I instruct.

Caleb is too forceful and shreds the vein.

"Bulldog, suction, clamp," I snap reflexively while grabbing the vessels before they retract out of view. The field is welling up with blood and Caleb momentarily freezes.

"Caleb, suction now; I have to be able to see," I whisper urgently. I have seconds to get control before the bleeding becomes a major problem.

Out of the corner of my eye, I see my boss scrubbing in. But before he can finish, I grab the vein with my instrument and advance the cannula into position. "Now tie down the silk," I tell Caleb.

One cannula is in and the bleeding is controlled. I can feel my heart thumping in my chest. I remind myself that no one in the room can detect my momentary fright. I take a deep breath to slow my heart rate. "Arterial cannula next," I instruct.

We get the second cannula in and then it's time to go on circuit. In a series of swift, fluid movements we remove the tubing clamps and I announce, "Going on ECMO—now." There's a rush of blood as Nia's oxygen levels start to climb. "Good color change," I reassure the team. The monitor shows her oxygen levels are now perfect. Nia's lungs can rest while the ECMO machine does the work for her. For the moment, she lives to fight another day.

I retreat back to my office to finish my notes. I try to call Nia's mother to tell her everything went well, but the line is dead now. The nurses say she still hasn't shown up to the hospital. She'll probably lose custody if she never comes. The whole thing is heartbreaking. I know I'll be stalking Nia's chart all night to follow her labs. I'm invested in this baby: we're her family for now.

Any feeling of victory is fleeting. The idea that an otherwise healthy baby requires ECMO for Covid is terrifying. I thought this thing wasn't supposed to affect children as severely. At least, that's what the CDC has been telling us. The data is still very early, but the latest report I've read says that fewer than 2 percent of reported Covid cases have occurred in patients less than eighteen years old. But that's just the cases we know about. The studies from China have also suggested that few children have gotten sick with symptoms or required hospitalization. But their early data on Covid being a disease of the elderly are also turning out to be inaccurate.

Sparing children was supposed to be the one consolation of this wretched virus, and I'm not sure that's turning out to be the case anymore. Every time I think I'm beginning to understand how Covid works, I learn a new way it's starting to screw us over. Some people seem to think that it's the great equalizer—attacking both the rich and the poor. But it's simple to see that those living in poverty have the worst of it by far. There's no escape for the New Yorkers huddled into crowded housing conditions or shelters.

I decide to take a walk outside to clear my head. I zip up my fleece all the way as I step out of the revolving door into the damp April air. I think about everything this moment should have been. These last few months were meant to be the capstone of my surgical training—one final push to really flex my surgical muscles and prove to myself and my attendings that I'm ready to operate independently. And even though I handled the ECMO cannulation on my own, I feel completely shaken and humbled by Covid. I don't feel like a strong, competent surgeon. I feel like every day I am just scrambling to try to keep myself, my team, and my patients alive. And I'm terrified that each day at the hospital will be the day I catch Covid myself—or, worse, that I'll carry it to Connecticut and infect someone I love.

I plop onto a bench. The bridge of my nose is throbbing and I need a break from my N95. I feel the cool rush of air as I break the seal and let myself inhale the outside air. But across the street I hear a deep, rattling cough. There's a man huddled under the awning of a bank. He's much older than I am and wearing a thick black down coat. He's just sitting there on the ground, head in his hands, in the posture of utter defeat. He's holding a cell phone. Ambulance sirens blare in the distance, surely headed toward our emergency bay. He looks up and briefly we lock eyes, staring at each other for a moment, both expressionless. He looks away first, checking his phone. Then he hoists himself up, ripping another huge cough, stares at me one last time, waves his hands at me dismissively, and then trudges off around the corner and out of sight.

SUNDAY, APRIL 26

The health costs of depression and physical inactivity that are resulting from so many people being holed up indoors are getting some media attention. People are aware that Americans are languishing in front of screens, Zooming, bingeing movies, surfing on social media, or spending too much time eating, drinking, and getting high. But there's another symptom of pandemic malaise that's familiar only to emergency room doctors and surgeons: people are showing up in the ER with all kinds of dangerous objects ingested or inserted into their orifices.

Rob is now being called into the emergency room at least twice a week to remove foreign bodies from people's rectums—everything from sex toys to glass bottles. We joke that there should be a public service announcement: "Please be responsible with what you put up your rectum!" It makes us laugh, but the last thing healthcare workers and hospitals need right now is for their resources to be further strained by regular removal of items from people's nether parts.

Meanwhile, on the pediatric side, I'm getting calls every day from the children's ED about toddlers who have swallowed a coin, a Lego part, a marble, a magnet, or anything else they could get their hands on. This was a common enough pediatric emergency pre-pandemic, but it seems to me to be worse right now. And when the children are Covid positive, it adds a new and difficult wrinkle to the story.

Tonight, the ED has called me about Z., a one-year-old who swallowed a penny about three days ago and is now gagging, coughing, and refusing to eat. An X-ray shows the penny is stuck high in Z.'s esophagus.

To remove a coin from a baby or toddler's esophagus, we typically have to put them to sleep, place a breathing tube into their trachea, and then fish out the coin or toy with a camera. That's all complicated enough. But Z. has just tested positive for Covid. So have both of his parents, who are here with him. This means that getting the penny out will entail significant risk of Covid exposure for everyone involved.

When I go to check on Z., he's coughing all over the place. It's a chaotic mess trying to figure out where to put everyone during the procedure to reduce exposure risk. When we bring Z. up to the operating room, there's no place for his parents to wait. The emergency room staff ends up sending them to wait in a car in the parking lot behind the hospital. This is certainly not the humane treatment we were trained to give worried family members pre-Covid, but the virus makes every aspect of our usual care more complicated. The game of avoiding overly risky exposures means that once-simple pre- and postoperative protocols now require going through a labyrinth of considerations.

I try to keep my focus on the logistics of the procedure and getting all the correct instruments together. We are short-staffed again overnight and I have to put together my own OR table if I want everything to be right, something our capable nursing staff used to do. We all don extra masks and eye protection.

My camera and a grasper go into the esophagus smoothly. I'm able to find the penny and wiggle it clear from the spot where it's been sitting for a few days. However, I find a shallow divot in the mucosa of the esophagus where the penny was lodged. It's midnight. Z. should be okay but I want to keep him at the hospital overnight for monitoring.

The nurses push back: there's no space to watch a Covid-positive baby; all the rooms are full. The head nurse tells us the baby would have to go to the PICU because it's the last available pediatric bed in the hospital. But the PICU protests—appropriately, because they're vastly understaffed tonight and no one wants to use one of the precious isolation rooms for this baby who just needs overnight monitoring.

I understand, but there's nowhere else for this poor child to go, and we're all being held hostage in the operating room as a result. I start to get frustrated. We just need to find a unit with a bed and a team willing to take care of him.

The anesthesia team wakens Z. from his sleep and he begins wailing and shrieking, exposing everyone in the room to a thick veil of Covid droplets. I immediately get on the phone with the hospital supervisor to figure out what we can do. I also call Z.'s parents to assure them the procedure has gone well and apologize for all the delay and confusion. Finally, I march up to the PICU and beg them to take baby Z. for the night. At last they agree but say they need at least an hour to prepare the room and reorganize their staff. I accept. It's the best we can do.

I return to the surgical team to find Z., now fully awake, trying to crawl off the operating room table. Molly, one of our best OR nurses, scoops Z. up in her arms and begins to rock and shush him. It's such a brave decision. We aren't supposed to cradle Covid-positive babies this way, and Z. isn't even wearing a mask. But this is a frightened baby. Molly saw that he simply needed to be held. She strokes the back of his head while swaying with the natural grace of an experienced mother. Immediately, the baby starts to calm.

Once Z. is set up in his room in the PICU, his parents are allowed to join him. They all sleep there until they are able to go home the next morning.

MONDAY, APRIL 27

Dr. O. is extubated! Not only that, he's neurologically intact. Jane tells me he's already giving orders to the residents. It's some of the best news I've heard in weeks.

I don't want to get ahead of myself, but it's a moment of hope that gives me the confidence to believe there will be an end to this awfulness. And it's coming at a time when there is additional reason for optimism. New York is successfully driving down new infections and hospitalizations. We are learning more and getting better at combating the virus at the hospital. Covid isn't sneaking up on us anymore. We know where to look for it.

Yet, even as things are starting to look more hopeful at the hospital, I am plagued by worsening insomnia, and nightmares in those few hours when I'm able to sleep. I've been having a recurring dream in which I'm standing in the emergency department with no PPE, surrounded by screaming children and their parents. The children are all coughing up blood, choking and gasping for air. Their parents are yelling at me to help. But in the chaos I am paralyzed. Like a statue, I stare blankly at them and my feet are pinned to the ground by a heavy magnet. I am helpless and worthless and scared.

When I'm awake at night, depressive thoughts invade my mind. Seeing my kids move on with their lives in Connecticut, being separated from Rob, and experiencing the sense of futility at the hospital over the past weeks have left me wondering if there's any point in my existence. *Maybe everyone would be better off if I were gone*, I sometimes think. I once revered my profession, but now I don't know if I can bear to keep up the façade of altruism. We aren't heroes; we're just sitting ducks, stupid enough to sign up for a job that we thought was about helping people.

We have all been so quick to congratulate ourselves for our selfless bravery. But the truth is that we lost so many lives unnecessarily. It's a spectacular failure. And it's not even really the fault of the doctors or nurses or even the hospital. We are just part of a larger, very broken system. Seeing how broken it is makes me want to run far away from this job and medicine. It would be such a relief to disappear.

People are sick of the preaching: stay home; wear a mask. I want to keep pushing that message, but it will be an uphill battle to encourage everyone to maintain vigilance in protecting themselves and their families and neighbors as things improve. Many people are still in total denial. They don't appreciate that we'll continue to need social distancing. Everyone just wants to get on with their lives. They don't want to hear that until we get a vaccine, we can't get anywhere close to pre-Covid, in-person social interaction.

I can't seem to eat anything. Any food I try to eat tastes like plastic. I look like a bag of bones underneath my scrubs. I have a history of anxiety and have had a handful of true panic attacks in my life that first started in medical school. After a particularly bad breakup during those years, I went on a low-dose antidepressant that effectively numbed my grief. I know I should probably go back on meds now, but I worry about having to disclose any mental health diagnoses as part of my future job credentialing and licensing. I don't even know how I would get in touch with a psychiatrist right now. I could just ask a friend for a prescription, but that would technically be illegal and jeopardize their license. Plus, they are all too overwhelmed with people suffering even worse than I am, just trying to cope with daily life. I am resigned to trudging through the next few weeks until I can figure that out.

WEDNESDAY, APRIL 29

Jason is a four-year-old who comes to the hospital at the end of April. His mother tells us that he caught a bad cold in March. They eventually took him to a hospital in Brooklyn, where he was given a breathing tube in the emergency room. Soon after, his oxygen levels began to plummet, and he was transferred to us. We put him on ECMO right as he arrived.

He's testing positive for the flu but negative for Covid. The extent of the damage to Jason's lung makes me doubtful, though. His lung has developed necrosis and it's weeping out of his numerous chest tubes. The testing is still so unreliable, and part of me thinks this has to be Covid. I've never seen regular flu do that to a child. He reminds me of Angie. He was perfectly healthy before this hospitalization. But I don't want to throw conjecture on this tragedy. I keep it to myself.

Jason's mom tells us that he lives for the cartoon *PAW Patrol*. His favorite character is Chase, the police officer pup. He likes to run around the apartment capturing "bad guys" and Jason's dad pretends to be caught in jail. I imagine Jason at his home and then at the playground, a bundle of energy.

On Wednesday night, Jane and I get the call that Jason is crashing. We rush in to try to save him. His heart is damaged beyond recovery from the stress of his illness. He's on ECMO and the body can only sustain so much. We put in another ECMO catheter, this time in his groin, but an hour later there is still no improvement. Jason is maxed out on everything. We watch as his blood pressure ominously starts to dip on the monitor.

After the commotion dies down, Jason's mother pulls up a chair next to his bedside. He still has a pulse, but barely. She starts stroking the top of his head and I can feel myself begin to lose it. I hurry to the stairwell to sob.

Jason's mom knows before all of us are ready to admit it. Her baby is gone.

The ICU attending calls the time of death five minutes later, at 2:16 a.m.

THURSDAY, APRIL 30

As this brutal month comes to a close and the picture in New York continues to improve, there is much talk about what our new normal will look like.

The surgery department chair's email update strikes a cheerful note:

> With great relief, today I watch the cruel month of April come to an end, and look forward to better things. What better new beginning than to think about scheduling patients for surgery? A large quantity of deferred benefit is waiting to be delivered, to those for whom it's not already too late.

I'm with him. I'd like to get back to the business of routine surgery again. But it doesn't seem to me like we're anywhere close to that. When we open the hospital back up in full swing, there will be huge pressure to make up for the financial losses and canceled operations. We'll be working twice as hard after already having gotten pummeled. They're even talking about doing routine cases on Saturdays and Sundays to play catch-up. That's not much to look forward to.

"Is it getting better?" everyone I know who isn't a healthcare worker asks me with a tone of desperation. *Well, kind of.* The doors of the emergency room are not being battered down like they were a few weeks ago, but a huge number of critically ill patients are parked in makeshift ICUs on ventilators. And they're not moving anywhere quickly.

What concerns me more: even as a physician, I don't have a good grip on how New York City is going to tackle the enormous task of widely testing our population, contact-tracing future positive cases, and reopening parts of the economy in a risk-stratified fashion. We need to build up a huge public health infrastructure that frankly doesn't exist in order to safely accomplish any of those tasks. Governor Cuomo assures us that we're sorting out how to get back to normal, that it's coming, but I want details of how and at what cost. Short of a vaccine, I am not very hopeful that any semblance of normalcy is on the horizon soon.

Whatever our new normal will look like, there *are* things about it that I believe are here to stay, and that I appreciate. I feel pride that doctors and healthcare workers are being honored and given a platform to speak their truth in ways they never were before. Suddenly everyone stuck at home wants a glimpse inside the world of the hospital. We are the microcosm of what the rest of the world will look like, the world's thermometer. Physicians have claimed a voice in the national media like never before, and CNN has medical guests on nearly every hour. Many of my peers and friends now have bylines in major news outlets. Valuable unsung heroes such as respiratory therapists and environmental services are getting recognition too.

But it took tens of thousands of Americans dying in the span of a month to get us here. Every pretty blue-check Twitter verification of a doctor brings me mixed feelings of hope and also queasiness. Our new spotlight has come at an enormous expense.

And as my friend Adrienne the ICU nurse reminds me, it's far from over. There have been so many deaths in her unit recently— several each day. Most of these patients are still dying alone. But she describes one that was unique, profound, and a reminder of something closer to what death in a hospital is meant to look like. The ICU made an exception for a patient whose daughter works in the hospital. The daughter and her mother were allowed to say goodbye to her father, who had been on a ventilator for weeks battling severe Covid.

Despite some of the best ICU care in the country, he took a turn for the worse. By the second week in April, all of his organs began shutting down. Death was imminent.

Adrienne is training several nurses on the floor who are new to ICU care. When the daughter and wife started wailing as they watched their father's and husband's heart wind down to a halt on the monitor, the new nurses turned to Adrienne with grief in their eyes.

"I can't handle the wailing," one of the new nurses said.

"No, honey, that is a beautiful sound," Adrienne replied. "That is what it is supposed to sound like when your world is falling apart."

The wailing gave Adrienne her first taste of "normal" in weeks.

FRIDAY, MAY 1

Maria—one of the best nurses not only in the pediatric surgery department but the entire hospital—is quitting.

This is part of an understandable but worrying trend. In the first weeks of the pandemic, so many of the best and most experienced nurses left, especially those who didn't need to keep working and were ready for retirement but had continued showing up because they loved taking care of children so much. Just about anyone who didn't need the paycheck to survive was out. With these senior nurses gone, the hospital lost a huge amount of institutional knowledge and expertise. A new crop of traveling nurses and fresh graduates are populating the floors and operating rooms.

Their lack of experience shows. It isn't their fault; they just don't yet know the particularities of each surgeon's preferences. Dr. H. only uses Vicryl sutures. Dr. S. likes to start his morning cases at

7:00 a.m. on the dot—or else. Dr. V. is notorious for getting hangry if he doesn't get a break by 2:00 p.m.

Maria is the same age as me and one of the greats. Originally from the Dominican Republic, she's a fantastic pediatric surgery nurse who knows all the tricks in the OR. Throughout my fellowship, she has been my go-to when I need to find some obscure instrument or a new tray. She never gets flustered and she loves working with the surgeons. Whenever there is a new nurse in the OR who needs to be trained, Maria is the one who supervises. She's the only one who remembers how to put together the bronchoscope the correct way. I always knew it was going to be a good day if I saw on the schedule that I would be in the OR with Maria.

But, like much of our OR staff when the pandemic struck, Maria was redeployed to the adult side to help in the ICUs.

"In the beginning it was okay because it was crisis mode," she tells me over a cup of coffee outside of Starbucks, where we have a few minutes to talk. She felt pride in showing up as part of the team taking care of the sickest Covid patients. She felt dignity and honor in her work as a nurse. But as the weeks dragged on, she started to feel like she was being taken advantage of. "The doctors don't even come in the room anymore, and we have to manage so many drips, all day long," she says. The staff numbers dwindled and Maria found herself performing the job of two or three nurses. "I was environmental services, tech, respiratory therapist, nutrition, and more on any given shift," she told me. It wasn't sustainable. Even worse, as more nurses quit, Maria's supervisor expected her to train and assist the traveling nurses who came to help fill in the ranks.

The sense of camaraderie among the nursing staff was eroded by the blatant unfairness in workloads and assignments. Often the traveling nurses were taking home much higher pay than the staff nurses, whose median pay annually was not that much more than the national annual median of $75,000. Nurses' wages have been stagnant for nearly twenty years, according to the Census Bureau, while physicians, surgeons, and pharmacists have seen large increases. Registered nurses experienced "little or no gains in median earnings since 2000," according to a bureau report.

For Maria, pay was not the main driver of her discontent. "One morning, I had two patients crashing on me at the same time," she tells me. "I called for help and nobody came. They were too busy re-intubating another patient across the unit." That's when she knew she was done. Maria actually worried that she could risk losing her nursing license if a patient coded or died on her watch. "What they're asking of us over there, it's not safe," she said, shaking her head. "I'd rather be home with my kids."

She has two children at home, doing school over the computer. Her mother has been helping out here and there when she can, but mostly Maria has been relying on her younger sister for childcare. Her daughter's grades have been falling, and the tug of motherhood is pulling her home.

Not for an instant do I blame Maria for quitting. Everyone is cheering on "healthcare workers" as an all-encompassing team of medical personnel in the pandemic, but nurses are the ones truly fighting night and day. Nurses are the real front line. They spend by far the most time at the bedsides of Covid patients. They get stuck with pretty much all the dirty work and little reward. Nurses often have the least autonomy over the makeup of their shifts and are increasingly at the whim of inexperienced or distracted doctors who don't fully process the risk and the stress of the nursing role.

"I can make twice as much or more if I go work for an agency," Maria reminds me. "But at this point I'd rather just be home or work at Starbucks; at least I'd get a discount." She laughs.

"Do you think you'll ever come back to hospital nursing?" I ask. "You're so freaking good at it."

"I don't know, CG. I need a long break from this hellhole."

Though I'm sad to see Maria go, part of me also feels proud of her and her fellow nurses for standing up for themselves. My hope is that this wave of resignations might give our hospitals a necessary jolt. They will eventually have to own up to the way they undervalue their nursing staffs and reckon with placing a disproportionate burden of the Covid work on them.

SATURDAY, MAY 2

After a draining day of surgery, I'm in my office wrapping up my last few notes and orders before heading home for the evening. My calves feel tight, swollen, and achy from standing all day. My neck pulses with the strain of hunching over sick babies on the operating room table in an attempt to make them whole again. I pull off my scrub cap and even my scalp feels tired from being constricted all day.

I'm heading home but I'm on call tonight and it's my habit to check the emergency room docket before leaving. There's nothing worse than leaving only to have to turn around within minutes, called back for an emergency, in my case usually for a ruptured appendix. So I scan the list of complaints on the ED board and if I see a note of "abdominal pain, nausea," I'll swing by the ED to see if it looks like an appendectomy is likely to be in my near future.

It's been eye-opening to see how the list of complaints has evolved. Before the pandemic, there was always a mix of the usual childhood illnesses: croup, strep throat, earaches, asthma, as well as injuries from accidents and falls. Then in March and April it was all fevers, shortness of breath, coughs. Now the complaints have changed again. "Suicidal ideation—10 years old. Toxic ingestion—9 years old. Violent outburst at home—8 years old."

The mental toll this pandemic is taking on children is immeasurable. Substance abuse, suicide, psychosis, eating disorders—all of the mental health issues of adolescence have skyrocketed, and we're seeing major episodes of depression and suicide attempts in younger and younger preteens. Domestic violence is skyrocketing. Across town, my friend tells me that an entire children's surgical ward has been converted into a pediatric psychiatric unit.

I can't blame any of these kids for the way they're feeling. In high school I remember thinking a bad test score was the end of the world. A friend's impulsive rejection would gut me. With Covid, the preteens and teenagers of the world have had to watch the sudden collapse of our social fabric. Powerless and isolated, they have stood by and watched the adults around them struggle to make sense of the madness. They've been torn from their friends and their schools. It's developmentally appropriate for teenagers to discover their sense of identity away from their parents; they can't do that right now. Instead, they're being forced into suffocatingly close quarters with them.

As I scroll down the ED board, I come across the listing for room 13. "Right lower quadrant pain, nausea, vomiting—14-year-old girl." That sure sounds like an appendix, so I decide to go see the patient before I leave. I walk down to the ED and peek into the room through the glass doors without being seen. The girl, Zoya, is lying quietly in the dark while her parents sit and scroll on their phones. I ask the ED resident nearby if she knows the situation and if they were planning to call surgery.

"It's a strange story," the resident tells me. "She actually had her appendix out a year ago."

Weird. Well, there's a good chance I can head home after all.

"Did you guys get any imaging? Sometimes there's a remnant stump that can get reinfected," I remind the resident.

"She had a CT of her abdomen and pelvis already: stone-cold normal. So are her labs. The radiologists can see the staple line of the old appendix and they're sure there's no stump."

"Got it. Okay. Sounds like you won't need me! You know how to find me if you do."

It's still early, and I decide to take the subway home for the first time in weeks. Covid numbers are on the downtrend. I am wearing a mask, and ridership is still sparse. Plus, my Uber charges are getting insane.

The express train moves swiftly, and in twenty-three minutes I'm downtown. I walk from the subway stop to my apartment and notice that people are beginning to mingle at the new outdoor setups at the bars and restaurants. The weather is getting warmer and New Yorkers are reemerging. A group of twenty-somethings are gathered in front of the vintage-looking speakeasy across the street, holding plastic cups filled with take-out cocktails. They're maskless. They're laughing loudly, happily, optimistically.

The sight of these revelers is a relief as well as an irritant. I can understand how desperate everyone is to gather again. And I guess it's safe enough to gather outside, where transmission is much less likely. But it also feels like a slap in the face to watch them be so carefree. They probably all have remote jobs and get to loaf around in sweatpants most of the day while those of us at the hospital are working overtime. I've always worked punishing hours, but the consolation prize before this was how much I loved my job. There's a lot less to love right now. Our ICUs are still packed with dying patients. Jane just lost a woman our age in the ICU this morning. "Her kids were just a few years older than Jayden and Maya," Jane told me in her office. Her eyes looked gone as she said it. There's nothing like that experience to remind you of your own mortality.

Before I open the door to my building, I hear the group across the street discussing whether they can have a pizza delivered right to the bar. A pair of them start dancing on the sidewalk between the tables. *Are you kidding me? Don't they understand the gravity of what the city has just been through? How can they be dancing?*

And then I catch myself, struck through with guilt at judging them. *Why not seize the moment while the weather is warm? Why not grab life by the horns again and demand that we all begin the march back to normalcy—whatever normal means anymore?*

224

If there is one cold hard truth I've learned from crisis, it's that the world moves on, impervious to your despair. You can either sulk and choose misery or find a way to climb your way back to the land of the living. I haven't had a cocktail since January. Maybe I'm just jealous and need a drink.

I go upstairs, shower, fix myself a bowl of my go-to canned lentil soup, but am too tired for a drink by that time so I go to bed. I think of the suicidal nine- and ten-year-olds in the emergency room. *How will the world ever convince them that the ship will right itself? Maybe the vaccine will come sooner than we think?*

I honestly have no idea what the timeline of Covid will look like. *Will lockdowns be a cyclical necessity for weeks or months or years?* We have very little way of predicting, and the messaging from the CDC is either confusing or nonexistent. Learning to cope with uncertainty is becoming an essential survival skill.

I jolt awake at 2:00 a.m. to check my phone, worrying that I've missed an urgent call from the hospital. I know I have to slow my racing heart before there's any chance of falling back asleep. I start doomscrolling Twitter. More political vitriol. More desperate pleas for prayers for loved ones hospitalized near and far. Darkness upon darkness. I switch to TikTok for funny dancing videos. Gen Z knows how to distract themselves from the apocalypse.

SUNDAY, MAY 3

I wake up in the morning and trudge back to the hospital. When I print my list for the day, I notice that room 13 is still occupied by the same fourteen-year-old girl, Zoya.

Not good.

I go to the emergency room and find her nurse. "How come room 13 didn't go home?" I ask.

"She still says she has pain all over. Can't keep anything down."

I need to examine her myself. Even though the imaging is negative, I don't want to miss a surgical problem if she has one.

When I walk in the room and introduce myself, her parents say they're relieved to talk to a surgeon. I explain that I'm going to take their daughter's history and do a physical exam if that's okay with them, and they agree. Zoya is lying down with her eyes closed, wincing.

"Are you in pain, Zoya?" I ask.

"Yes, every day," she replies.

Zoya's parents tell me a more detailed version of the story I got from the ED resident last night. About a year ago Zoya had her appendix out and everything seemed fine. She was a freshman in high school. She had a close group of friends and excelled at her schoolwork. She was captain of the freshman field hockey team and she loved to play the flute. But things changed for this happy teenager when Covid hit. She began having mood swings and then panic attacks. Her pediatrician prescribed a low-dose antidepressant but it was impossible to get an appointment with a therapist for regular counseling. By the time May arrived, Zoya was barely leaving her room or eating meals.

"She says her stomach hurts—all the time," her mother tells me.

Zoya has been seen by multiple doctors. She's had multiple CT scans, MRIs, ultrasounds, and X-rays. She's had upper and lower endoscopies to see if there's any problem with her intestines. She's been seen by a gynecologist. All of Zoya's studies came back normal; all of her doctors cleared her. After months of chronic pain, no one has any answers.

"We think someone needs to take a look with surgery," Zoya's mother explains. They were at their wits' end. "It's the only thing left to do. The last doctor said this was all in her head, but look at her: she's in real pain."

Cases like Zoya's are some of the hardest ones for surgeons. Much of our radiologic imaging has become so sensitive that we can pick up very small abnormalities. When a patient complains of chronic abdominal pain and everything turns out negative, it can be a long, frustrating journey for the patient, their parents, and their doctors. For many girls and women in particular, pain that we cannot obviously explain through abnormal imaging or labs gets brushed off as "supratentorial"—basically, a trick of the mind. The pain these patients feel is just as real as any appendicitis. The cure, however, is much more elusive.

Some doctors specialize in the treatment of "functional abdominal pain," which usually involves a system of trial and error with diet changes, medications, allergy testing, and relaxation techniques. Sometimes a simple elimination diet does the trick. Other times, children suffer for years on end without relief. Researchers still have fairly poor understanding of the causes of functional abdominal pain.

As I examine Zoya, I look carefully for any hints as to the cause of her pain. She barely speaks five words to me and is visibly anxious, with her hands tightly gripping the sheets of the stretcher at her sides. I can't find anything in my examination. She has no tenderness. Pressing on her belly doesn't hurt her at all. But Zoya is in pain. I take more history and even interview her separately, with her parents out of the room, trying to make sure I'm not missing anything. We're seeing more and more children at the hospital who are victims of abuse at home. It doesn't always manifest as cuts and bruises. Sometimes vague, unexplainable pain can hint at psychological distress. But Zoya is clear with me that she feels safe at home and with her parents. I leave her room to talk more with the emergency room doctors, who agree there is no reason to suspect abuse.

"Frankly, I think it's all in her head," one of the ED residents says.

"Maybe, but people don't ask for surgery unless they are truly desperate," I point out.

I go back into Zoya's room and explain that another team of gastroenterologists will come to see her, since there isn't an obvious surgical problem. I assure Zoya and her parents that I'll come back later in the day to check on them, but by the time I return in the afternoon, Zoya has been discharged. The family got sick of waiting around and were sick of being treated like their daughter's pain was imaginary.

I'll never know what was truly causing Zoya's pain, but I can say for certain that people are suffering as a result of shortcomings of our healthcare system and lack of mental health resources in particular. I am meeting teenagers who are unable to attend school due to crippling anxiety over Covid. Nearly every patient over the age of eleven has "anxiety" listed as an active problem in their chart right now. There are children who have been assaulted so violently by relatives that they wind up intubated in the ICU.

My kids are too young to really grasp the true depth of the pandemic and are largely spared from the effects of crippling anxiety. But they dearly miss their friends and teachers, and I worry whether all the experiences they couldn't have during Covid will amount to longer-term problems.

TUESDAY, MAY 5

The chair's update email is illuminating.

> Bringing my epidemic saga full circle, yesterday an ELISA assay
> [a Covid antibody test] revealed that I have anti-coronavirus
> antibody. In late February I was sicker than I have ever been,
> with relapsing fever and racking cough. When short of breath
> at night the sounds in my lungs made me think of bagpipes
> thrown to the ground. Assuming I had an unusually bad
> influenza, I carelessly worked every day as usual. As far as I'm
> aware, I didn't infect others, but who knows? If true, thank my
> gift for social distancing.

Clearly, Covid was here in February. I think back to the week
at Eloise's nursery school when everyone was sick. I was never sick
in February but Rob and Eloise both had terrible fevers just after

Presidents' Day. I think back to Angie. I think back to all the careless, maskless running around we did and the foolish choice I made to attend that last birthday party for Eloise's friend that Sunday in March. I still can't understand why or how Covid could kill so many people and manifest as a bad cold in others. It feels so arbitrary and unfair.

The chair's email makes me desperately wish to get us all tested for antibodies. In some ways it would be a great relief to know my children have already been exposed and recovered. But we also have very little understanding of the long-term effects of the virus on the immune system. For now, I have no good reason to justify testing my family. I have no choice but to follow the flimsy public health guidance and carry on with work.

WEDNESDAY, MAY 6

A video showing the fatal shooting of Ahmaud Arbery is everywhere. The pain of Black and brown communities in the United States is front and center in our minds at the hospital and beyond. My friend Imani, a Black senior surgery resident in Boston, posts her outrage on Facebook and it captures the anger I can only begin to imagine as a white woman.

Imani was my intern on the liver surgery service when I was a senior resident. She was so quiet the first time we rounded together. I took pride in earning her trust and eventually drawing out her witty sarcasm by the end of her rotation. Watching her mature into her role as a senior resident and begin to really use her voice is inspiring. But as she states in her Facebook post, the police shootings, on top of the toll Covid is taking on people of color, are wilting her spirit.

CORNELIA GRIGGS

She writes:

Instead of just being fatigued from having my daily life upended by this virus, I have to see it ravage Black and brown communities because of the unjust system we propagate in this country. On top of that I have to watch cops bully and beat Black and brown faces for not social distancing (many who couldn't if they wanted to) and watch them hand out masks and joke and laugh with their white counterparts across town. Let's not forget the videos of armed protestors—who were so quick to say blue lives matter—disrespect cops and get ZERO PUSHBACK, yet when we peacefully protest we get riot gear. Now you want to bombard me with videos of a modern day lynching and remind me that in fact my life and people who look like me still don't fucking matter. You want to know what it's like to live in my shoes? Do you see now why my views of this country and the world are so pessimistic? Do you now see why I have zero tolerance for racism, bigotry, sexism, and any other -ism you can define? I do not have the capacity to "accept" the ugly, nor should I be asked to. I smile out of defiance. I laugh out of resistance. I exist for the revolution. I may not live to see the change I demand—but that won't stop me from trying. If my message is too much for you, that's your problem. Feel free to step aside. I don't have time to wait. My people are dying and I refuse to stand by and watch them be thrown away.

I know I can't begin to really understand the pure rage the current climate for Black Americans is provoking. The best I can do is closely follow and amplify the voices of my Black friends and colleagues. I promise to be a supporter and to validate their lived experiences.

THURSDAY, MAY 7

With streaming tears of relief, I watch a video, taken yesterday, of Dr. O. coming out of his room in a wheelchair and mask and down to the main lobby of the hospital to send a message of thanks to the team who has been caring for him. "My name is Dr. O. I am one of the surgeons here. I am supposed to be on the front line helping others, but I myself caught the Covid pneumonia and it was really, really tough. I was on the ventilator for two weeks and even ECMO a few days. But thanks to my colleagues and thanks to God, I was able to survive. I am still in the hospital. I'm not able to walk independently yet."

He goes on to talk about how thirsty he's been since he was extubated and how the nurses give him ice cubes that quench his thirst and help him talk again.

"I'm just always joking with the nurse, 'This is a whole new world. I can even sing a song!'"

Then one of Dr. O.'s favorite residents, who is sitting at the piano in the hospital lobby and happens to be an amazing piano player, launches into the opening bars of "A Whole New World," from the Disney movie *Aladdin*. Dr. O. has a microphone in hand. From his wheelchair, he sings the entire song. The audience joins in with him. His voice is still audibly raspy from all the time he spent with a breathing tube, but our Superman is back. It's hard to even capture how uplifting and utterly adorable the whole scene is. I will treasure this. No matter how disappointed I am in so many of the ways that people have acted during this pandemic, examples like this of the unbreakable human spirit will keep me going.

SUNDAY, MAY 10

I'm called over to the ED to see two children with something we are now calling post-COVID inflammatory syndrome. Both of them arrive in the emergency room with terrible belly pain and a rash. Both of them recovered from Covid a few weeks ago. The surgery team is consulted because there is concern about a possible abdominal emergency. Both children's symptoms mimic those of a disease called Kawasaki syndrome. Both of the kids are put on high-dose steroids in an attempt to quell the inflammation ravaging their bodies.

There's a statewide health alert that has everyone on edge, especially on the children's side of the hospital. There are reports of an outbreak in Britain, and now there is a sense of alarm here. There are supposedly more than eighty cases of this multi-inflammatory syndrome in kids across New York City. According to the news, at least five children have died as a result. Though we were already aware in the hospital that children were not always being spared from

Covid and that the supposed silver lining of the wretched disease wasn't so simple, the wider public is now taking notice.

Meanwhile the governor is talking about a phased reopening of New York State. Some regions upstate could be open in just a few days. I understand the need for reopening the economy. The U.S. Department of Labor figures show that, in the last eight weeks, more than 36.5 million Americans have filed for unemployment. It's hard to even wrap my head around what that means for tens of millions of American families. With what seems like the worst of the surge behind us, I can feel the swell of eagerness to get back to the lives we had before this fearsome virus had everyone locked in their own homes. But I am also terrified of reopening without enough testing and what it will mean for hospitals. The pop-up ICUs are just starting to shut down. If we open up restaurants and other venues too soon, we will land right back where we were, with swarms of patients gasping for air knocking down the doors of emergency rooms.

TUESDAY, MAY 12

I'm catching flak from another surgeon on Twitter—this time from a woman I have always admired, even adored, which stings.

I posted that our PPE situation is still nowhere close to "normal" and she responds that "normal" means despicable waste strewn in our oceans and the bellies of whales. She writes that she's been using the same N95 for a month and is antibody negative, so therefore I should "get on with it." In other words, shut up, stop complaining, and move along.

I respect this surgeon not only for her technical ability but for her refusal to take bullshit from anyone. Clearly, she thinks I'm the bullshit now. *Ouch.* I'm not a proponent of waste by any means. Protecting the environment is obviously important. But when it comes to protecting our healthcare workforce, having clean, safe PPE is essential.

The experience is making me question once again whether social media and medicine are simply not a good mix. What I thought was a fairly innocuous post has now ruined my day and cost me the respect of someone I admire.

Our traditional mode of writing manuscripts in medical journals is slow and outdated. I've always preferred writing for a broader, nonmedical audience. Social media seems promising because it allows a large platform and quick dissemination of knowledge and exchange of ideas. But you also open yourself up to creeps, critics, and haters when you go on Twitter. After years of being more of a lurker on social media, I'm still learning how to navigate using it in a professional capacity.

It's hard for me to accept that I'll never please everyone with my message. I know that a lot of people with Twitter followings eventually find themselves embroiled in drama or full-on cancellation. But maybe I still take things too personally to have a big platform. You need a thick skin to do Twitter well. I'll probably never get there. And if my posting on Twitter is somehow creating the illusion that I'm not doing my day job, as the other surgeon suggested a few weeks ago, I'm not okay with that. I'm still working twice as many hours as most of the people coming to criticize me. But I'm also catching the attention of my future bosses in Boston, most of whom don't use social media at all. One of these surgeons called me today to warn me that people have taken notice of my new swell of followers, and it's causing some concern. It's clear that my future posts will be monitored.

I won't stop being a whistleblower when I feel it's important. But I also know that the next phase of my career is one where I will be vulnerable to a higher level of scrutiny. A misstep on Twitter could cost me my career. So I am making a commitment to myself to stop posting as much. Losing the respect of surgeons I admire isn't worth it to me. What I do post, I will keep professional and more nuanced, if that's possible on Twitter.

Outside, two residents are tossing a football in the garden. It's a glorious spring day and the sun is shining brightly. I can almost forget that the morgue is still packed and that more of the mobile ones will probably be needed. But the arrival of warm weather means I am that much closer to graduation and, with it, freedom from Covid hell in the hospital. At least until I get back to Boston, where I hope things will be much better by the fall, when I start my new job.

SUNDAY, MAY 17

—

FRIDAY, MAY 22

According to the Johns Hopkins tracker, we surpassed 1 million Covid cases on May 17. It feels like the truly terrible milestone it is.

On the eighteenth, a very sick baby named Molly comes into the NICU. Molly's mother, Gia, stands vigil at her bedside every moment that she can. It's her first child, and like so many NICU mothers, she pinned her hopes and dreams on this baby. When Gia went into extremely premature labor at twenty-three weeks, she was freaked out and heartbroken. Molly survived delivery but is tiny, like a fragile baby bird.

I'm called into the NICU to monitor Molly's belly closely because the team caring for her is worried she could be getting a serious intestinal infection called necrotizing enterocolitis. Taking care of preemies is extremely humbling work. Sometimes they are more resilient than you can imagine and other days they seem to crash on a whisper. Molly's little belly is swollen to the size of a grape.

Her skin is translucent. Over the following days, I keep checking on her. She seems to be holding her own.

On Wednesday the twentieth, Kay and Nathan fully move out of their apartment. Like so many young families who once lived in the city, they are bound for the suburbs for good. Maybe they always were, but it feels like Covid has hastened a move for them and many others with young children. Rural life has a newfound appeal after this harrowing spring in the city.

Kay left the BabyBjörn bouncy seat that I lent her out in the hallway, too afraid to actually come inside my apartment. I don't blame her. We say goodbye from opposite ends of the hallway. We both start crying and mock ourselves for once thinking we would be hanging out at the pool together on the Fourth of July.

It's the end of a magical little era, living side by side and co-raising our kids in solidarity. We do an "air hug" goodbye and then she is in the elevator. I have no idea when I'll see her again, if ever. I'm feeling a mix of jealousy and sympathy. We are both burned out by the demands of Covid and motherhood.

Jane and my other friends in healthcare are in a similar boat. We're trying to juggle distance learning for our kids, sorting out safe and reliable childcare, enforcing mask and cleaning protocols at work and at home, dealing with endless questions from friends and family, managing the stress and worry of Covid risk to ourselves and our loved ones—all of which leave no time to process the trauma of working on the front lines. Moms everywhere are at their breaking point already, with no relief in sight. No one is sure how long their kids will be out of school. Even if they do open schools in the fall, I am totally torn about what I will do with Eloise and Jonah when it comes time to decide whether or not to send them. Luckily, I still have the summer to sort that out.

On Friday morning, I go to check on Molly and she seems to be doing well.

"She's having a good day today." I smile at Gia. "Little girl is a fighter."

But in the afternoon she takes a dramatic turn for the worse. Molly's belly suddenly swells with air. Something has perforated. We have to get permission to do a risky emergency procedure at Molly's bedside to try to save her. We need it fast.

Gia is distraught and can't decide what to do. Every minute counts. She asks me to call her sister Cara, who is a nurse at a hospital in New Jersey. Cara is not allowed inside because of visitor restrictions due to Covid, but I know she often comes and sits outside the CVS Pharmacy across from the hospital, just to be near her sister. She answers. She's there.

"Cara, this is Dr. Griggs. Your sister needs you now," I tell her.

Taking pity on the situation, one of the aides helps me sneak Cara up the back elevators of the hospital and into the bathroom outside the NICU. There, we give her a pair of our scrubs so she will blend in. I bring Gia to the bathroom and they embrace. I step out and let them have their time together.

Small acts of rebellion like this against the hospital's strict Covid rules allow us to preserve some semblance of humanity. Being robbed of our ability to practice compassionate care takes a toll on everyone. Helping Cara be there for her sister on the worst day of her life feels right, and I'm grateful to the aide who risked her job to make it possible.

After two minutes, Cara and Gia emerge from the bathroom and give us permission to go ahead with the procedure. They know it is a high-risk scenario, but to do nothing means almost certain death.

I go to Molly and open her belly. The damage is already too severe. Too much of the bowel has already started to die from overwhelming infection. In spite of our efforts, she's slipping away from us.

I etch Molly's name into the back of my OR logbook. She joins the little cemetery that I keep there of patients who have died during my training years here in New York.

TUESDAY, MAY 26

In the wake of yesterday's brutal murder of George Floyd, our country is facing a crisis of social unrest in the name of justice. I reach out to Imani, and she shares her thoughts on the day's events with me by email:

> By the time my alarm went off, I had probably been awake
> for about half an hour. I was staring at the ceiling with a pit
> in my stomach, replaying the images of the knee on his neck,
> listening to his cries echo in my head. I had watched a man die
> last night. I watched him scream for his mother in fear, and I
> listened as bystanders screamed at the cop to get up and called
> for help that wasn't coming. Sleep escaped me for most of the
> night, and in its place were fits of tears, waves of rage, and a
> sense of helplessness that overwhelmed me. George Floyd's
> death sapped what little feeling of togetherness the pandemic

response had garnered in me. The COVID-19 pandemic exposed the holes in the public health system as it ravaged poor and underserved communities. There was a magnifying glass on health disparities and their role in the disproportionate number of deaths of thousands of Black people from COVID. Being a Black physician was already complicated as I grappled with how best to support my community while dealing with the general anxiety carried by all healthcare workers about what was to come. But George Floyd's death was the proverbial straw that broke the camel's back for me. His death was a reminder my Blackness will always be the greatest immediate threat to my life and the lives of those who look like me.

I did not want to get out of bed, let alone work for the next 24 hours. The last thing I wanted, or needed, was to be surrounded by people who were seemingly unaffected by the murder of another innocent Black person. But I did what was expected of me. I got out of bed and got dressed. While walking the dog, I allowed myself just a few more moments of open grief before steeling myself against the emotions as best as possible before heading to the hospital for my shift. Learning how to mask feelings is a lesson many Black people, especially women, learn at a young age. We are conditioned to understand that displays of emotion that make those around us uncomfortable are unacceptable. By the time I walked into the hospital, I had composed myself and was able to return pleasantries with colleagues as we ran into each other in the hallway. But as expected, there were no words or even acknowledgment of the death of George Floyd. As the day went on, interacting with my colleagues became more difficult. I began to tune out the workroom gossip and stories of their pandemic hobbies or zoom happy hours. My grief bubbling just below the surface constantly threatened to expose me and drove me to retreat to the call room where I could be left to my thoughts. The physical and emotional isolation of the pandemic and now the murder of George Floyd left me grappling for something solid to hold on to and steady myself.

We keep the conversation going, and Imani tells me just how much it hurts her that she feels she's getting "radio silence" from her colleagues. She calls it "deafening." She says:

I began to regret my decision to pursue a surgical career. Not only did I pick a field that was systematically built to exclude me, but I was also at an institution that still has not come to terms with its own ugly past with slavery and the oppression of Black people. I could not see how spending hours toiling away in the ivory tower was going to amount to any significant change for my community. I wanted nothing more than to hang up my white coat, walk out the doors, join the protestors in the streets, and never look back. At least then I could yell, and someone would hear me, see me, and see the pain and heaviness I was carrying. I wanted the world to not only see but feel the pain that so many Black Americans carry to this day as we continue to be excluded from society and left to defend our humanity. I was at war with myself, at war with my country, and at war with the silent killer that was COVID-19.

Imani did protest, taking to the streets of Boston, "yelling for justice and speaking life into the names of the Black lives stolen from us." And she also took to social media, both her own and mine for a time, after accepting my offer to take over my Twitter account. She tells me:

I no longer cared if my words made people uncomfortable. Black people were dying because of an unjust system, a system that we are all complicit in when we stay silent. There was no room for silence, no room to sit by and allow the comfort of my peers to be prioritized over the lives of Black people. With every post, I found a new depth to my voice.

Through the combination of protest and writing, she says, "I was able to release the coils of tension."

THURSDAY, MAY 28

One of our ER physicians has died by suicide.

Lorna Breen is her name. It's all over the national news. I didn't know her, but I work with many people who did. We must have interacted at some point in my training because she was one of the directors of the emergency room. She was forty-nine with no reported history of mental illness. She was an avid traveler.

In the *New York Times* article detailing the distressing circumstances of her death, her father says, "She was truly in the trenches of the front line." She had described to him the awful scenes she was witnessing as an onslaught of patients flooded into the emergency room. Her father's assessment was stark. "She tried to do her job, and it killed her."

Apparently, Dr. Breen had caught Covid, then returned to work less than two weeks later. But something was still off, and she went to her family's home in Charlottesville to recuperate. The article described Dr. Breen as seeming "detached" to those around her. Her family "could tell something was wrong." She died by suicide in Charlottesville.

Our entire medical community is shaken, not just at our hospital but around the city and the country. Dr. Breen's death is a reminder of how much we've all been through and the toll it's taking on us. It's a reminder that we are all vulnerable. As much as each of us would like to think "that couldn't or won't happen to me," there is very little reason to believe with certainty that it's true. In so many physician suicides, which are frighteningly common in comparison to people in other professions, we are quick to mentally distance ourselves from the victim. We rationalize the irrational by pointing to a history of mental illness or other extenuating circumstances that give us a thin explanation. The truth is, most physician suicide is impulsive and leaves families wondering why and how this could happen to someone so successful, so loved, so wonderful. The truth is Lorna Breen is all of us.

—

The human toll of Covid goes far beyond those directly felled by the virus. Dr. Breen *is* a Covid death. She's also a heroic physician in every sense. To honor her, we must promise to do better for patients and providers alike.

No one knows the right way to process and honor what we have all just survived. Doctors, nurses, and other healthcare workers will continue to become victims of the mental anguish, trauma, and distress that accompany living through this unprecedented tragedy— that much I know. I am so sick of the words "unprecedented" and "unimaginable" but I still find myself using them almost daily. Today I am making a promise to myself that as soon as I graduate, I will make the time and space to work with a therapist, to talk through everything I have seen, heard, and felt over the last excruciating months. Writing this journal is helping, but I know that it is hubris to think I can process this all without professional help.

FRIDAY, MAY 29

The pandemic situation really *is* improving. Some people in the hospital who were redeployed are now returning to their normal job functions. More and more space is opening up in the operating room, allowing us to take more cases. The strokes, heart attacks, and broken bones that had somehow evaporated are showing up again.

Preventive care had been moved to Zoom or telephone appointments, and, predictably, there are consequences that we're now starting to see as people show up for in-person examinations. Raquel, whose worsening abdominal pain and cramping has been managed by phone for the last three months, is only sixteen. Her doctors assumed that her symptoms were related to anxiety, but Raquel is precipitously losing weight and can barely keep any food down.

Finally, she's able to come into the hospital for a CT scan. My friend Laura, a pediatric oncologist, calls me as soon as she gets the results. The scan shows a melon-sized tumor wrapped around Raquel's kidney and nearby organs.

"This one is gonna be a doozy," Laura tells me. The tumor is enormous, atypical, and invasive.

I walk over to the pediatric oncology division to meet Raquel and her parents. Though she's a teenager, Raquel appears childlike. She is extremely small and thin. Her veins bulge from her spindly arms and her skin has an unhealthy, transparent quality. She's always been a picky eater, her parents—who are warm, with thick Brooklyn accents—explain, so it took them a while to notice that she was losing weight. I ask the raven-haired girl about her symptoms. She can barely speak, so she just nods her head yes or no.

When I finish my interview and exam, Raquel's mother looks at me and asks desperately, "Did we catch this too late? I should have brought her in sooner."

I take a breath before I respond, not wanting Raquel's mother to hear the catch in my voice. "The important thing is that you're here now, and we're going to do everything to get this mass treated as quickly and as safely as possible."

My heart aches thinking of the overwhelming sense of guilt Raquel's mother is feeling. But it's not her fault. It's not anybody's fault. We are living in a broken system with a virus that has crippled our ability to deliver care.

The oncologists and I plan out the battery of tests we'll give to Raquel to figure out if the cancer has metastasized. The tests come back a few days later and show that it has. We organize a group conference to discuss whether the tumor can and should be removed surgically, and we determine that the answer is yes. We book Raquel for a massive operation to hopefully remove the whole mass. I block off an entire day for the case.

On the morning of the operation, I meet Raquel in the pre-operative area. She has brought a stuffed raccoon, and the nurses adopt the tone of voice they usually use with younger kids. She doesn't seem to mind.

I hold Raquel's hand as we wheel her into the operating room and move her onto the operating table. We've decided to start with an epidural to help with the pain that will come from the large incision we need to make across the left side of her chest wall and abdomen. I rub her shoulders as the anesthesiologists struggle to get the catheter between the tiny vertebrae of her spine. She winces with each additional poke, grinds her teeth, but never once complains.

I try to distract her. "What's your favorite place to go on vacation?" I ask.

"Disney," she whispers.

———

The team finally completes the epidural and Raquel goes off to sleep while I'm still holding her hand. I make a silent wish for her to dream of Disney while we work to extricate that nasty tumor from her insides.

We start the operation with the incision across her left side. We find the tumor. It's big but proves simple to free: I easily cut it away from Raquel's kidneys and other vital organs. I'm feeling optimistic. Then we see a new section of the tumor. It's completely wrapped around the lower part of Raquel's aorta and the arteries that supply blood to her pelvis and leg. If we injure the arteries, she could lose a huge amount of blood or even a limb.

Like an angry wad of hardened gum, the tumor refuses to come free from those arteries. I finally have to start cutting away at it with our sharpest pair of scissors and a fresh blade. One slip of the hand and we'll be in major trouble, because we have only tenuous control of the vessel that is tunneling through the tumor. We slice at the tumor millimeters at a time while sparing the essential arteries. The surgery takes hours.

To our incredible relief, it's successful. But while we're confident we got the mass in her abdomen and chest, we know that the cancer has metastasized in such a way that it's possible she has cancerous nodules in other places as well. Raquel could still have a long battle ahead.

I can't help but wonder what would have happened if Raquel was seen in person at her first complaint. Would her pediatrician have felt the hard mass growing on her left side? If not for Covid, could she have been diagnosed in time to prevent the aggressive spread of her tumor? I'll never know.

There could be millions of other cases out there that are, if not as uniquely rare and dangerous as Raquel's, consequential nonetheless. How many moles that went unexamined are evolving into malignant melanomas? How many skipped mammograms, and colonoscopies, and other routine evaluations, will lead to cancers taking months or even years longer to diagnose?

More subtle but just as insidious is the likely effect Covid will have on our country's obesity crisis. All the sedentary screen time and overeating that we're learning has been extremely common will translate into more pounds, more heart attacks, more diabetes, and more liver disease down the road for so many Americans.

It will take decades for us to really know what the full public health impact of this pandemic truly is.

MONDAY, JUNE 1

I've been to two protests in downtown Manhattan and Brooklyn in support of the Black Lives Matter movement so far, both totally peaceful. While I do worry about everyone gathering in the streets and what it could mean for Covid numbers, I know that this moment demands outrage and demonstration. So today after work I decide to join another near Union Square. Still wearing my scrubs, I meet my best friend Eliza there. She's a public defender and many of her clients are young Black men sitting in prison on Rikers Island, awaiting trial for petty charges after being unfairly targeted by police.

Despite the histrionic media coverage and reactions from many outside of New York, the protestors have been overwhelmingly peaceful. It's the police who have acted with brutality against unarmed Black civilians. But as Eliza and I are marching tonight near the corner of Fifth Avenue and Fourteenth Street, with the sun setting, the scene around us erupts into chaos.

At first we're not sure what's happening, but soon we see a Foot Locker being looted right across the street. We hurry to get out of the center of the crowd. We're not afraid of the other protestors, but sirens are wailing from every direction. We know that the police are on their way and things around us are about to get more turbulent.

The crowd is attempting to disperse in every direction. Eliza and I turn down a side street but have barely made progress when a group of young teenagers starts yelling and running toward us.

"Hey! Are you a nurse? Hey! Do your damn job! People are hurt over here," they say.

"What do you need?" I ask.

Then I see a teenage boy with his T-shirt wrapped around his hand. There's a small puddle of blood in the street at his feet.

I approach, telling him that I'm a surgeon and asking him to show me his wound. He unravels the shirt and reveals a long but shallow laceration across the back of his hand. He refuses my suggestion to seek care at an emergency room, so I offer to clean his wound in the street. His friends have gathered supplies from a CVS Pharmacy around the corner. I clean and bandage his hand, he thanks me, and he and his friends head to Brooklyn while Eliza and I split up and go to our apartments downtown. The sky is getting dark and people are setting off fireworks nearby. New York City is officially under curfew. Outside the looted shoe store, dozens of stray sneakers are scattered across the empty street.

The store owners near my apartment are boarding up their shops.

It looks like a zombie apocalypse is underway. MINORITY OWNED, someone has written in Sharpie across the plywood covering one store's windows.

"No justice, no peace. No justice, no peace." The protest chants echo in my head as I try to fall asleep.

FRIDAY, JUNE 5

It's Eloise's nursery school graduation day. Diane, Eloise's teacher, has sent all of the kids little royal blue satin caps and gowns and instructions for the ceremony, which include moving the cap's tassel from left to right. I can't tell if Eloise is excited. It's virtual, of course, and for her it seems like just another morning of trying to sit still in front of her iPad in Connecticut. That's been harder for her lately, my mom says.

I'm working, so I miss the live ceremony. But as soon as I get home, I pull up the recording. Eloise pops up on-screen in her own little digital window, surrounded by her fellow Sharks. She looks so adorable in her cap and gown—and proud too. It's nice to see all the kids together at one time on the screen, even though they're physically separated. As Diane leads the ceremony, my mother floats in and out of the picture, trying to keep Eloise standing and focused.

Diane has also planned out a group dance performance. My mom holds the iPad camera up to capture Eloise as she dances alone for a minute in the dining room. Then Eloise gives up. It makes me sad to see. I know that she loves dancing and would have had a great time doing the routine with her friends in front of a live audience. I've signed her up for ballet classes in Boston in the fall, but whether they'll happen is anyone's guess.

Next up in the ceremony is a long slideshow of pictures of the kids, set to schmaltzy music. Tears roll off my chin through the majority of it. There are pictures of the kids from the beginning of the year, pre-pandemic, and they all still look like babies to me. They're playing in the little kitchen, running around the rooftop gym, hugging each other. In almost all the pictures of Eloise she's with Titus, her close friend at school, who used to live a few blocks from us. Eloise and Titus were taken to school together every morning, and when my mom would pick them up in the afternoon, they would often persuade her to take them to the ice cream shop across from school before squeezing onto the subway. My mom misses Titus too. Eloise and Titus have had some remote playdates but it's just not the same. I'm going to call Titus's mom over the summer and see if it's possible to get the little lovebirds together at the beach.

I've missed so much of Eloise's school life because of my work. I never even got the chance to read to the class. Every other parent did it pre-Covid. I thought I would get a chance later in the school year. So much for that.

When the slideshow ends, Diane and the assistant teacher, Carrie, say something special about each Shark. They praise Eloise for being a great friend and for her humor. I'm so proud of her but also grieving all the sweet moments the students, teachers, and parents have lost to Covid.

MONDAY, JUNE 8

—

THURSDAY, JUNE 18

Things continue to get better over the weeks of mid-June. Though a steady trickle of patients still comes through the emergency room every day with a cough and fever, Covid numbers and deaths are plummeting. The morgue trucks leave the hospital and don't come back. People begin to talk about the surge in the past tense as we collectively agree that the worst is behind us in New York City.

With graduation coming up for me and Fred, our ECMO fellow, the whole pediatric surgery department decides to gather on June 18 for an outdoor dinner in Westchester at my program director's house. Jonah is in the city with me. The pediatric practice where he's a patient has started to allow occasional in-person visits again, and he's here for his two-year physical. I decide to bring Jonah with me to the dinner.

Gathering as a group—illicitly, by the hospital's current rules—feels strange but nice. It feels important. We sit at a picnic table on my program director's deck. He has a brand-new puppy named Maverick, a Rhodesian ridgeback who is floppy and adorable and bouncing with puppy enthusiasm. I can understand why so many of my friends have bought or adopted dogs during the pandemic. Maverick injects a dose of pure happiness into what's initially an otherwise semi-awkward social situation. One of the surgeons I work with jokes that if one of us has Covid tonight, the entire department is going down. We all laugh nervously; there is some truth to it.

The dinner is the first time in months that Jonah is around adults other than my parents and a babysitter. He is normally chatting away and bubbly, but when he sees these new adults he goes practically mute and clings to my side. Though intellectually I know this is perfectly normal behavior for a two-year-old, the anxious-mom part of my brain worries that isolation has affected Jonah's long-term development. He hasn't had any of the toddler activities and classes that we signed up for to help with his socialization. And he's still too young to engage meaningfully with anyone on-screen.

The effects of social isolation on my kids is a constant worry. Eloise is typically a social butterfly who loves to give hugs, even to children she's just met. In these past months I've trained her to shut down those physical, affectionate instincts, doubling down on lessons about physical boundaries, good germs versus bad germs, and so on. Am I programming my children to live in fear? I don't feel like I have another choice.

Despite being a doctor, I have never been a germophobe. I

ascribe to a healthy microbiome parenting philosophy and allow a five-second rule when a cookie or piece of candy hits the ground. I always accepted that every cold and flu season my kids would be exposed to a number of circulating viruses and we would cope with some Tylenol, Pedialyte, and a few missed days of school. When Eloise was a baby, toddling around at eye level with Magic, our golden retriever, I never worried if she caught a quick lick to the face or lips. But the unknowns around Covid make it much harder for me and other parents to accept any risky exposures right now. The wave of Kawasaki-type infections related to Covid was particularly scary and makes me fear that there could be further autoimmune implications of the virus in children down the road. I want to do everything possible to protect them. So I've become much more vigilant about all kinds of hygiene. I can't even look at a playground without visualizing the slide, the ladders, the monkey bars, all teeming with germs.

———

Parenting in a pandemic is a continuous exercise in worrisome choices. I get it that many parents are fed up with isolating their children, but I think people are going too far when they argue that prevention through isolation and social distancing is worse than the disease. It's especially frustrating to me that some people refuse to wear a mask or put one on their children. We still don't know the long-term effects of Covid on the heart, brain, or immune system. The mask, a simple prevention strategy, has become politically charged, mainly across party lines.

While things are better in New York, across the Sunbelt cases are still climbing. I hope they can at least learn from our mistakes. We know our enemy much better now. But if other hospitals and cities across the country fail to respect how quickly a Covid surge can cripple a local healthcare system, more unnecessary deaths are inevitable.

SUNDAY, JUNE 28

—

SUNDAY, JULY 19

Usually, the pediatric surgery department celebrates the graduating fellows with a fancy dinner party hosted at a restaurant or at the home of one of our attendings. Speeches and toasts and roasts are the norm. For Jane's graduation last year, I spent two weeks perfecting my speech, looking for that happy medium between humor and sentimentality. We both wore killer dresses and got our hair blown out. We joked that the attendings wouldn't recognize us. It was probably the first and only time my team saw me in makeup.

As fun as Jane's graduation was, I'm comfortable in the knowledge that it's too risky to do one this year. I'm not very sentimental, a product of being raised in my family. My mother cut up her own wedding dress and fashioned it into a Halloween costume when I decided I had to dress up as an angel one year. I skipped my medical school graduation and took the week to go on a hiking trip. Of all the things Covid has taken from us, I'm not terribly disappointed at the thought of passing on my fellowship graduation. After nine years of surgical training and nearly five months of Covid, I'm beaten down and bedraggled. My reserves of idealism about the medical profession are just about crushed. The last thing I want to do is put on a pair of heels and force a smile.

But throughout the weeks of late June, my chief insists. He's sentimental and refuses to let me leave without taking a night to commemorate the achievement. Training the fellows and shaping the future of the tiny niche field of pediatric surgery is a pillar of pride for the attendings. Over the past two years I've logged more operative cases than during my five years of general surgery residency in Boston. So I don't argue when I'm instructed to save the date—July 19—for an outdoor dinner in Midtown. It's going to be held at a Greek place where the head of our program knows the owner and we'll have free, if socially distanced, range. I emailed my family at the end of June to warn-slash-invite them—and gave them all a free pass to decline.

Rob and my mother decide to join. The rest of my family understandably decide to avoid gathering over a meal. On the day of the dinner, I straighten my hair, put on a light blue floral sundress, and make myself vaguely presentable. It's a sweltering evening as we approach the restaurant's makeshift outdoor dining tent. All of the surgeons from my department come, and I give a short speech expressing my deep gratitude to each of them for training me. My program director gifts me a small blue box from Tiffany with a silver key ring. My mentor hands me a plaque that says: "If you're not having fun, you're probably not doing it right," a corny joke he likes to crack in the OR. My chief presents me with a framed photograph of the children's hospital set against the Manhattan skyline. Jane gives a short roast and gifts me a pearl necklace—a symbol of grit and grace, she says.

We laugh, eat, and drink good wine, and for a brief moment we all pretend that Covid isn't a thing anymore. But one of my bosses hangs back a bit from the group. She's on maternity leave with a newborn at home and I appreciate that she's ventured out of the house to give me a proper send-off. When we're on our way out, she smiles at me gratefully when I pull back from the hug I'm about to initiate. We mothers understand. I do hug some of the other fellows and embrace Jane, my faithful work spouse, though. It feels wonderful.

I let gratitude wash over me when I'm back at home, reflecting on the night. No one in my family has gotten Covid so far. New York is beginning to come back to life. I love my colleagues and will miss them. We've come through this war together. I'm about to start the life I've dreamed of as a pediatric surgeon. I have the rest of the summer in Connecticut to play with the kids, exercise, and go to the beach. No more city and no more hospital. Rob will come down on weekends.

Battling Covid as a trainee has made me question nearly everything I believed about the medical field. It's made me confront my own mortality. Before the pandemic, I imagined that I would be a terrible soldier should I ever have to fight in a real war. Now I know that I'm capable of risking harm in service of others day after day. I've found in myself a steely kind of reserve that comes from confronting risks and making strategic calculations day in and out. While living and working in the middle of a crisis, I discovered the ability to compartmentalize fear. I learned to function in survivalist mode.

Maybe I still can't handle a real battlefield—who knows?—but I'm pretty sure I can get myself through other terrifying scenarios if I have to. At the very least, when the next doomsday scenario arises, I'll be a handy companion.

EPILOGUE

Looking back at the period I've written about in this book, it's striking to realize that the feeling that the pandemic unfolded overnight is in fact practically true. It was on January 30, 2020, that Covid-19 was declared a Public Health Emergency of International Concern by the World Health Organization. At the time, the official death toll was 171. By the end of the year, it was nearly 2 million—and due to the drastic underreporting of deaths in 2020, that's almost certainly an underestimate.

Many people feel that they want to put as much physical and mental distance between themselves and the time covered in this book as possible. That's understandable. Like everyone else, I'm tempted to want to move on with my life. And thankfully, much of life has gone back to something near normal. But the truth is, as I write this in spring 2023, the latest *New York Times* tracker suggests that there are still over 20,000 new Covid cases and 250 deaths every day in the United States—once again likely an undercount, as many states are not reliably tracking or reporting. Just yesterday I learned about a vaccinated, boosted patient younger than I am who is fighting for their life in our ICU.

These individual cases still send chills down my spine. Taking a step back, life inside the walls of the hospital where I worked—in fact, inside any hospital in the country, and likely the world—will never be quite the same again. The worst part about working in healthcare since the start of the pandemic has been the mass exodus of so many brilliant, dedicated doctors, nurses, and other professionals from the clinical practice of medicine. Not only do we miss their skill sets and personalities, but the level of understaffing at hospitals has made the job of caring for patients indescribably harder.

Most of the time, I still believe I have the best job in the world. Even on some of the darkest days of the pandemic, I felt truly privileged to be working and helping during what I certainly hope will have been the most severe health crisis of my lifetime. I think my intuitive sense that I was living through a historic moment in healthcare was also one of the reasons I was motivated to write it all down. It helped me to process the trauma I was witnessing and living through as it happened.

When people meet me and learn that I'm a surgeon, they often say something to the effect of "I could never do that." But what most of them really mean is that they would never *want* to do that. Because many people have the skill and brainpower to become a surgeon if they decided it was the thing they wanted to do most in the world. When I signed up for medical school and residency, I, like most of my generation of doctors, had no idea we were signing up to combat a massive global pandemic. This is why I'm continually inspired and motivated by a new generation of students who are applying to medicine and nursing and other healthcare professions despite what they witnessed over the last three years. This new cohort of healthcare workers is something fearsome. They are bringing much-needed demands for change with them. At the hospital where I work now in Boston, residents are organizing to unionize and advocate for better worker protection benefits and pay. A re-imagining of the old, punishing residency and training system feels long overdue. I do like to think our capacity for human compassion and empathy expanded during the pandemic.

The Covid crisis forced me to reevaluate and reconsider what I was made of not only as a doctor but also as a mother. I wanted to quit and take the next train to Connecticut and ride out the worst of the first wave at home with my children. Frankly, I chose my job over my children. I am still reckoning with what that means and what it says about who I am as a mother. At the time, the threat of being fired and stripped of everything I had worked for in my career was overwhelming. I couldn't look away from the opportunity to combat the biggest healthcare crisis of my time.

Now, Eloise, who is seven, and Jonah, who is four, are thriving. Eloise, a charmer by nature, is thrilled to be reading real books and laughing her head off over the antics of Beezus and Ramona. Jonah, doing all he can to rival his older sibling, has surpassed Eloise on the ski slopes and is bursting with pride. It feels like Rob and I are entering the golden age of parenting. We're in that magical window where hanging out with our kids is actually fun, they think we are great, and we don't need to bring a stroller or a diaper bag everywhere that we go. Weekends involve a lot of time outside together, dance parties, snuggling, and giggling. I can feel the presence of a near future in which Eloise will ditch us for her friends. It'll happen any minute now. I can't deny that it makes me question the value of hustling so hard in my career as an academic surgeon at Harvard. There are many days I hit my office, long after the sun has set, knowing I'm missing yet another bedtime. I still haven't found that mystical illusion of "balance" as a working mom. But I'm also not ready to give up on trying to solve some of our biggest problems in healthcare.

I'm still in school getting my master's degree in public health—a decision inspired by watching the government fumble the pandemic response so badly. I'm often left wondering what I was thinking. Most weeks, I struggle to find the time to complete my coursework. Sometimes on a Sunday night after we put the kids to bed, I have to stay up for another two or three hours completing my advanced logistic regression problem set homework. I silently question my own sanity and the life choices that brought me to this point. Who am I really trying to impress? Myself, I guess.

But then I remind myself: I'm here for a reason. Sadly, we're not really better prepared for another pandemic than we were in February 2020. One of my biggest motivators is thinking about how I can help improve the system to change that.

In addition to taking many emergency overnight calls every month, I am also working to launch a research platform in childhood obesity prevention and gun violence prevention. In the wake of the pandemic, we have seen an exacerbation of many chronic diseases in children as well as a major uptick in violence among young people. As an academic surgeon, I have the responsibility of trying to ameliorate these devastating social plagues.

I just keep showing up every day and chipping away at goals little by little—one assignment, patient, or case at a time. With any luck, those days will add up to a career that leaves future generations a little better off. Isn't that all any of us can hope for?

I hope that readers of this book will have found something to relate to in a story about human vulnerability, persistence, and how real bravery often looks and feels. As I learned, bravery isn't the obvious-looking thing we imagine it to be. It's something very mundane, even pathetic in the moment.

Bravery is feeding your children while holding on to your last bit of sanity during quarantine. Bravery is what essential workers did in showing up to work to keep the fabric of society intact. Bravery is social distancing from frail or elderly relatives for months or even years at a time, because we love them.

In college, I won a prize and was given an inscribed copy of *The Great Gatsby*—my favorite novel. During the depths of the pandemic, I sometimes began silently reciting its famous last line: "And so we beat on, boats against the current. . . ."

ACKNOWLEDGMENTS

I have to start by thanking my husband, Rob, who inspires me to be a better surgeon every day. I wouldn't have survived residency, fellowship, or any of it without you. Thank you for giving me the time and support to make this book happen. I love you madly. To Eloise and Jonah—you are my happiness and the greatest gift of my life. I can't wait to watch you grow and explore the world. I will always be your biggest champion.

To my parents—thank you for teaching me to dream big and with fierce determination. Thank you for being incredible parents and now grandparents. To Dad—you taught me to live a life of curiosity and learning. To Mom—the best Nana ever—I wouldn't have had the guts to write a book without your encouragement and frequent help. Thank you for believing in my voice from the moment I could use it. You'll always be my hero and my greatest role model.

To all of the friends and coworkers I interviewed for this book (you know who you are)—your testimony and experiences inspired me to share this story with the world. I have done my best to honor your bravery. Together I hope we can shape the medical field for the future—with more kindness, humanity, and imagination than we have currently.

To all the great surgeons and physicians who trained me—thank you for teaching my hands to heal sick children. Thank you to SS, JZ, EF, VD, and BMW, in particular. Thank you to all the great nurses and healthcare workers who taught me that good medicine is born mostly from compassion. Knowledge gets you only so far.

To my patients—you've taught me more than any book, any lecture, any lesson in school or training. Thank you for the privilege of caring for you.

To Will, William, and Lindsey—thank you for having my back, always, and rooting for me when Covid times got dark. Thank you to Jim and Jane for letting me hide at your house to write and sometimes nap in the hammock when the words wouldn't flow.

Thank you to all of the amazing helpers who make our household run—to Pam, Abby, Marsha, Anna, Estefania, and Claudia—you are my village and I love you for helping to raise my kids. This book was written in stolen moments you gifted me while being with Eloise and Jonah.

Thank you to Jen, Sandra, Claire, Eliza, Eneda, Cali, Liz, Danielle, Karen, Melanie, Imani, Denne, David, and all of my dear friends who have been cheerleaders throughout this process.

ACKNOWLEDGMENTS

Thank you to the MBC crew for being our social lifeline during those strange emergence months when we were learning to be with people again. Thank you to our amazing Charlestown neighbors for making Boston feel like home. Thank you to Steve, Bruce, Marjorie, Andrew, Arielle, Oliver, and Julius for being my bonus family!

Thank you to the pediatric surgery and ECMO team in New York who kept showing up even when it felt preposterously unsafe to do so. Thank you to the wonderful friends and strangers from around the world who shipped me masks when there were none to be found. Thank you to my current partners at MGH for always having my back. Thank you to my chief class and to all of the friends from near and far who texted or called to check in when NYC was flailing in the first wave. Thank you to Mei for help with the timeline and research.

Thank you to Suzanne Gluck, my agent, who saw something in my writing way back before I ever believed I could tackle a book of my own.

To Simon & Schuster—I am so honored to be publishing my first book with you. Thank you for believing in me and this project. Thank you to Max and Aimee for your patience and brilliance. Thank you to Jen B., Sally, Jen L., Caroline, Emily, Steve, Brigid, Hope, and everyone else who made the book possible.

Thank you to my readers and anyone who has followed my work and my writing. It's a privilege to write for you.

ABOUT THE AUTHOR

DR. CORNELIA GRIGGS is a triple board-certified pediatric surgeon. She completed medical school at the Columbia University College of Physicians and Surgeons, from which she graduated with Alpha Omega Alpha honors. She completed her adult general surgery residency and surgical critical care fellowship at Massachusetts General Hospital, where she currently practices. She is a graduate of Harvard College and earned a certificate in health policy from Harvard's John F. Kennedy School of Government. Her writing has been published in the *New York Times* and many top medical journals, including the *New England Journal of Medicine*.